Step 1

Step by Step Critical Care

Second Edition

Arun Kumar Paul
BSc MBBS DA MS (Anesth)
Ex-Professor
Department of Anesthesiology
Medical College and Hospitals
Kolkata, West Bengal, India

The Health Sciences Publishers
New Delhi | London | Philadelphia | Panama

Jaypee Brothers Medical Publishers (P) Ltd

Headquarters

Jaypee Brothers Medical Publishers (P) Ltd
4838/24, Ansari Road, Daryaganj
New Delhi 110 002, India
Phone: +91-11-43574357
Fax: +91-11-43574314
Email: jaypee@jaypeebrothers.com

Overseas Offices

J.P. Medical Ltd
83 Victoria Street, London
SW1H 0HW (UK)
Phone: +44-2031708910
Fax: +44 (0)20 3008 6180
Email: info@jpmedpub.com

Jaypee Medical Inc
The Bourse
111 South Independence Mall East
Suite 835, Philadelphia, PA 19106, USA
Phone: +1 267-519-9789
Email: jpmed.us@gmail.com

Jaypee Brothers Medical Publishers (P) Ltd
Bhotahity, Kathmandu, Nepal
Phone: +977-9741283608
Email: Kathmandu@jaypeebrothers.com

Jaypee-Highlights Medical Publishers Inc
City of Knowledge, Bld. 237, Clayton
Panama City, Panama
Phone: +1 507-301-0496
Fax: +1 507-301-0499
Email: cservice@jphmedical.com

Jaypee Brothers Medical Publishers (P) Ltd
17/1-B Babar Road, Block-B, Shaymali
Mohammadpur, Dhaka-1207
Bangladesh
Mobile: +08801912003485
Email: jaypeedhaka@gmail.com

Website: www.jaypeebrothers.com
Website: www.jaypeedigital.com

© 2015, Jaypee Brothers Medical Publishers

The views and opinions expressed in this book are solely those of the original contributor(s)/author(s) and do not necessarily represent those of editor(s) of the book.

All rights reserved. No part of this publication may be reproduced, stored or transmitted in any form or by any means, electronic, mechanical, photocopying, recording or otherwise, without the prior permission in writing of the publishers.

All brand names and product names used in this book are trade names, service marks, trademarks or registered trademarks of their respective owners. The publisher is not associated with any product or vendor mentioned in this book.

Medical knowledge and practice change constantly. This book is designed to provide accurate, authoritative information about the subject matter in question. However, readers are advised to check the most current information available on procedures included and check information from the manufacturer of each product to be administered, to verify the recommended dose, formula, method and duration of administration, adverse effects and contraindications. It is the responsibility of the practitioner to take all appropriate safety precautions. Neither the publisher nor the author(s)/editor(s) assume any liability for any injury and/or damage to persons or property arising from or related to use of material in this book.

This book is sold on the understanding that the publisher is not engaged in providing professional medical services. If such advice or services are required, the services of a competent medical professional should be sought.

Every effort has been made where necessary to contact holders of copyright to obtain permission to reproduce copyright material. If any have been inadvertently overlooked, the publisher will be pleased to make the necessary arrangements at the first opportunity.

Inquiries for bulk sales may be solicited at: jaypee@jaypeebrothers.com

Step by Step Critical Care

First Edition: **2005**

Second Edition: **2015**

ISBN 978-93-5152-540-0

Printed at : Samrat Offset Pvt. Ltd.

*Dedicated to
my loving wife Kanyakumari
and
daughter Sushmita*

Preface to the Second Edition

The second edition of the book *Step by Step Critical Care* has been expanded to some extent to include some important medical and surgical problems that arise in critical care unit. The object of the book remains the same to provide a concise yet comprehensive guide to critical care practice. It is designed to be used for rapid reference. The book is thoroughly revised and updated.

I hope that this edition will prove useful to the anesthesiologist in training and practice working in critical care units.

Arun Kumar Paul

Preface to the First Edition

The present volume *Step by Step Critical Care* provides a concise coverage of various aspects of critical care medicine. It is intended to provide a convenient and rapid source of information related to the subject. It is written in a simple and easy-to-understand format. Some major health disorders commonly encountered in critical care units are being selected to discuss in this volume. Each disease dealt in this volume is discussed with relevant practical aspects of the day-to-day care with particular reference to aetiology, pathophysiology, clinical manifestations, diagnosis and management. Various information and useful laboratory data are presented in accompanying CD ROM.

The book admittedly does not include discussion on all possible diseases treated in critical care units. If the readers find this effort worthwhile, it is my intent to develop it further in next editions.

I am thankful to Shri Jitendar P Vij, Chairman and Managing Director of Jaypee Brothers Medical Publishers (P) Ltd., who suggested the particular topic and actively co-operated at all stages of publication of this book.

I sincerely hope the presentation of this volume should satisfy the basic needs of all practising physicians, particularly those interested in critical care medicine.

Arun Kumar Paul

Contents

Chapter 1. **Respiratory Disorders** 1–28

Adult respiratory distress syndrome (ARDS) 1
Severe asthma: Status asthmaticus 5
Acute exacerbations of chronic obstructive pulmonary disease 8
Pulmonary embolism 10
Pneumothorax 15
Aspiration pneumonitis 20
Upper airway obstruction 24
Airway burn 26
Flail chest 27

Chapter 2. **Cardiovascular Disorders** 29–58

Acute myocardial infarction 29
Congestive cardiac failure 34
Acute pulmonary edema 39
Hypertensive crisis 44
Shock 46
Cardiac tamponade 53

Chapter 3. **Neurologic and Central Nervous System Disorders** 59–96

Head injury 59
Cerebrovascular accident 65
Cerebral edema 66
Status epilepticus 69
Poliomyelitis 72
Tetanus 74
Increased intracranial pressure 77
Brain death 82
Guillain-Barré syndrome 84

Coma 86
Traumatic spinal cord injury 90
Myasthenia gravis 94

Chapter 4. **Liver Diseases** 97–106

Acute liver failure 97
Chronic hepatic failure 102

Chapter 5. **Renal Diseases** 107–119

Acute renal failure 107
Chronic renal failure 112
Some nephrotoxic drugs 118
Diabetic nephropathy 118

Chapter 6. **Endocrine Dysfunctions** 120–133

Thyroid storm/Thyrotoxic crisis 120
Myxedema coma 122
Diabetic ketoacidosis 125
Hyperglycemic hyperosmolar
nonketotic coma 127
Hypoglycemia 130
Acute adrenocortical insufficiency 132

Chapter 7. **Temperature Illness** 134–141

Heat stroke 134
Malignant hyperthermia 135
Hypothermia 138

Chapter 8. **Poisoning** 142–159

Self-poisoning 142
Barbiturate poisoning 145
Salicylate poisoning 146
Paracetamol poisoning 147

Tricyclic antidepressants poisoning 148
Lithium poisoning 149
Narcotic poisoning 150
Poisoning with various tranquilizers 151
Organophosphorus poisoning 151
Alcohol poisoning 152
Carbon monoxide poisoning 154
Cyanide poisoning 155
Poisoning with amphetamines 155
Cocaine poisoning 156
Poisoning by toxic irritant gases 157
Poisoning with caustics 158

Chapter 9. **Cardiopulmonary Resuscitation** 160–168
Cardiopulmonary arrest 160

Chapter 10. **Fluid, Electrolyte, and Acid-base Disorders** 169–193
Dehydration 169
Pure water-deficiency 170
Water intoxication (excess) 171
Hypercalcemia 172
Hypocalcemia 174
Hyperkalemia 175
Hypokalemia 177
Hypernatremia 179
Hyponatremia 181
Hyperphosphatemia 184
Hypophosphatemia 185
Acid-base disturbances 186
Metabolic acidosis 187
Metabolic alkalosis 188
Respiratory acidosis 190
Respiratory alkalosis 191

Chapter 11. **Miscellaneous** 194–215
Disseminated intravascular coagulation 194
Acute pancreatitis 198
Drowning 202
Total spinal anesthesia 204
Transfusion reactions 206
Dengue 213

Bibliography 217
Index 219

Chapter 1

Respiratory Disorders

Adult Respiratory Distress Syndrome (ARDS)

Adult respiratory distress syndrome (ARDS) is a nonspecific pulmonary condition characterized by abnormal permeability of pulmonary capillary endothelium leading to progressive accumulation of fluid within the lung parenchyma and alveoli. Mortality is mostly due to multisystem organ failure and systemic hemodynamic instability over and above acute severe lung dysfunction. It is also known as shock lung syndrome, or noncardiogenic pulmonary edema.

The exact cause is not always certain, but the possible disorders predisposing to ARDS are as follows:
 1. Shock
 2. Sepsis
 3. Multiple injuries, lung trauma, and head injury
 4. Aspiration of gastric contents
 5. Near-drowning
 6. Smoke inhalation and burns
 7. Acute radiation pneumonitis
 8. Snake poisoning
 9. Fat embolism
 10. Disseminated intravascular coagulation (DIC)

11. Acute pancreatitis
12. High altitude, oxygen toxicity, and hypoxia
13. Severe viral or bacterial pneumonia
14. Overdose of heroin, methadone, etc.

Pathophysiology

1. Progressive accumulation of extravascular fluid within the lung parenchyma due to derangement of alveolar capillary permeability.
2. Excessive accumulation of fluid in the alveoli of lung leads to decreased pulmonary compliance, increased dead space ventilation, and increased intrapulmonary shunt fraction.
3. Hypoxemia is mostly due to:
   a. Hypoventilation
   b. Diffusion defect
   c. Mismatched ventilation—Perfusion
   d. Intrapulmonary shunt.
4. Hypercapnia is due to:
   a. Impaired CO_2 elimination due to decreased alveolar ventilation.
   b. Mismatched ventilation—Perfusion.

Clinical Features

1. Progressive hypoxemia, tachypnea, dyspnea, cough, sputum production, and air hunger.
2. Restlessness, confusion, somnolence, and coma.
3. Tachycardia, cyanosis, hypotension, hemodynamic instability, shock, and cold extremities.
4. Hypoxia, hypercarbia, decreased lung compliance, pneumonia, decreased breath sounds, wheezing, and rhonchi or gurgles.
5. Respiratory failure.
6. Multisystem organ failure.

Investigations

1. Chest X-ray:
   a. Pneumonia and atelectasis.
   b. Increased pulmonary vascularity, interstitial infiltration, opacities, white out of lung fields, and loss of lung volume.
2. Arterial blood gas analysis:
   a. Increased $PaCO_2$.
   b. Decreased PaO_2.
   c. Decreased pH.
   d. Alveolar arterial oxygen gradient (A–aO_2) becomes more than 20 mmHg.
   e. Ratio PaO_2/FiO_2 less than 200 mmHg.
3. Pulmonary function tests:
   a. Decreased total lung capacity.
   b. Reduced vital capacity and forced expiratory volume.
   c. Increased closing volume.
   d. Pulmonary wedge pressure — Low.
4. Total blood count.
5. Sputum culture.
6. Histological changes:
   a. Massive interstitial edema.
   b. Hyaline membrane.
   c. Loss of surfactant.
   d. Atelectasis.

Management

1. Ventilatory dynamics should be improved. Mechanical ventilation and controlled oxygen therapy are most vital. Endotracheal intubation and mechanical ventilation with positive-end expiratory pressure are most effective to minimize and open up the airway

and alveolar collapse, to decrease the intrapulmonary shunt and to improve overall V/Q abnormalities and to increase the functional residual capacity of the lung. It will alleviate hypoxemia. But peak end-expiratory pressure (PEEP) level needs adjustment to get the optimum benefit. PEEP may reduce the cardiac output and adequate measures and inotropic drugs may have to be used to prevent hypotension.

2. Monitoring of vital signs, blood gas analysis and central venous pressure (CVP) monitoring are essential. Pulmonary artery and wedge pressure needs attention.
3. Intravascular fluid volume should be maintained carefully. Crystalloid solutions may be used. Fluid overload should be avoided. Packed red cells or blood transfusion may be necessary.
4. Diuretics: Frusemide.
5. Dopamine to raise the blood pressure and to maintain adequate renal blood flow.
6. Steroid therapy is controversial.
7. Acid-base balance should be maintained according to blood gas analysis.
8. Extracorporeal membrane oxygenation may have some value in such cases.
9. Inhalation of nitric oxide 5–80 ppm may decrease pulmonary artery pressure and improve arterial oxygenation.
10. Treatment of the underlying cause as in cases of sepsis where broad-spectrum antibiotics should be given according to culture and sensitivity test.
11. Bronchodilators and mucolytic agents may often be helpful.
12. Careful nursing care, care of the airway, tracheobronchial toilet, airway clearance, and adequate

nutrition—Enteral or parenteral—All these are of vital importance for such critically ill patients.
13. Prognosis largely depends on:
    a. Underlying precipitating factors.
    b. Degree of ventilatory dysfunction.
    c. Degree and severity of hypoxemia.
    d. Degree of capillary leakage.
    e. Response on drug therapy and mechanical ventilation.
    f. Early detection and intensive therapy and care are essential to reduce the incidences of mortality.
    g. Mortality is mostly due to the effect of hypoxia, infection, systemic hemodynamic instability, and multisystem organ failure.

Severe Asthma: Status Asthmaticus

Status asthmaticus is a serious medical emergency and may be life-threatening, refers to a severe asthmatic attack, often refractory to usual bronchodilator therapy. Bronchial asthma is a respiratory disease characterized by increased responsiveness of the airways to various stimuli, reversible expiratory airflow obstruction and chronic inflammatory changes in the submucosa of airways.

Essential Pathophysiology

1. Release of some chemical mediators like histamine, immunoglobulin E, prostaglandins, etc.
2. Some abnormalities of autonomic nervous system regulation of airway tone causing imbalance between excitatory and inhibitory airway tone.
3. Widespread bronchoconstriction causing hypoxemia, airway narrowing, increased airway resistance, increased work of breathing, decreased vital capacity,

increased functional residual capacity, hypoventilation, hypercarbia, and so on.
4. Chronic airway inflammatory response resulting to emphysematous lung changes.

Predisposing Factors for Acute Attacks of Asthma

1. Inhalation of irritant gases, vapours, dusts, smokes, foreign substances, and antigens.
2. Ingested antigens.
3. Upper respiratory tract infections—Viral and bacterial.
4. Reflux of acid gastric fluid into the lower esophagus.

Clinical Features

1. History of asthma.
2. Difficulty in respiration, dyspnea, coughing, and wheezing.
3. Tachypnea.
4. Exhaustion, fear, and dizziness.
5. In acute attack, nasal flaring, respiratory distress, flushed, moist, diaphoretic skin, cyanosis, restlessness, agitation, progressive fatigue, wheezing, expiratory stridor, and so on.

Investigations

1. Total blood count.
2. Arterial blood gas analysis, hypoxemia, hypercarbia, and acidosis.
3. Chest X-ray.
4. Pulmonary function tests.
5. Electrocardiogram.

Warning Signs

1. Cyanosis.
2. Tachycardia and pulsus paradoxus.

3. Level of consciousness—Confusion and drowsy.
4. Breathlessness.
5. Inability to expectorate.
6. Sleeplessness.
7. Arterial blood gas analysis, hypoxemia, and hypercarbia.
8. Pulmonary function tests—Decreased. Forced expiratory volume in one second (FEV_1) less than 35 percent predicted.

Management

1. Adequate ventilation and oxygenation:
   a. Humidified oxygen.
   b. Mechanical ventilation.
2. Bronchodilator drugs:
   a. β_2-agonists, albuterol by metered dose inhaler. Salbutamol by intravenous (IV) infusion.
   b. Theophylline 5 mg/kg IV followed by 0.5–1 mg/kg/hr.
3. Anti-inflammatory drugs: Corticosteroids in high doses.
4. Correction of abnormal gas exchange:
   a. Acidosis should be corrected with hyperventilation or medications.
   b. Bronchospasm should be relieved.
   c. Monitoring of arterial blood gas analysis.
5. Care of the airway.
6. IV fluid infusion to correct dehydration.
7. Antibiotics to control bacterial infection.
8. Anticholinergics: Ipratropium may have some value.
9. Mucolytics: Acetylcysteine to liquefy and promote expectoration of mucus.
10. Emergency treatment of status asthmaticus should include:
    a. Repetitive administration of a β_2-agonist by inhalation or injection.
    b. Corticosteroids in high doses.

c. Intubation and intermittent positive-pressure ventilation (IPPV) in desperate cases.
d. General anesthesia with volatile anesthetic may be tried to produce bronchodilation on rare occasions when even aggresive drug therapy fails.

Acute Exacerbations of Chronic Obstructive Pulmonary Disease

In chronic obstructive pulmonary disease there is limitation of airflow secondary to either airway disease (chronic bronchitis) or destruction of lung parenchyma (emphysema) or both. There may be sudden progressive hypoxemia and hypercapnia in such patients resulting in acute respiratory failure.

Pathophysiology

1. Infection is the most common cause. In chronic bronchitis expiratory airflow is obstructed by mucous gland hypertrophy, mucous plugging and narrowing of the bronchial tree. In emphysema, dilatation of airspaces distal to terminal bronchioles and destruction of alveolar walls cause a loss of the elastic recoil of the lungs and reduce the expiratory airflow.
2. Progressive hypoxemia and hypercapnia.
3. Often related to smoking and urban pollution.

Clinical Features

1. History of productive cough and sputum for years.
2. Shortness of breath and fatigue.
3. Headache, restlessness, confusion, somnolence, and coma.
4. Dsypnea, tachypnea, and cough.
5. Cyanosis, tachycardia, diaphoresis, and arrhythmia.
6. Rhonchi, decreased breath sounds, and decreased lung expansion.

Investigations

1. Chest X-ray: Flattened diaphragm, increased anteroposterior chest diameter, bullae, hyperlucency, and hyperinflation of lungs.
2. Lung function tests:
   a. Vital capacity—Reduced.
   b. Total lung capacity—Increased.
   c. Ratio FEV_1 and forced vital capacity (FVC)—diminished less than 75 percent.
   d. Maximum breathing capacity—Reduced.
   e. Maximal mid-expiratory flow rate—Reduced.
   f. Residual volume—Increased.
   g. Functional residual capacity—Increased.
3. Arterial blood gas:
   a. Decreased $PaCO_2$
   b. Increased $PaCO_2$
   c. Decreased pH
4. Total blood count
5. Sputum culture.

Clinical Features Suggesting Respiratory Failure

1. Exhaustion and fatigue
2. Irritability, restlessness, drowsiness, and somnolence
3. Coma
4. Rapid shallow breathing
5. Diaphoresis
6. Cyanosis
7. Inability to expectorate.

Management

1. Reversible factors of the disease such as infection, bronchospasm, and heart failure need adequate attention and management.

a. Infection: Antibiotics.
   b. Bronchospasm: Bronchodilator therapy and steroids.
   c. Heart failure: Diuretics.
2. Sedatives, narcotics, and tranquilizers should be avoided as they suppress respiratory drive and cough.
3. Chest physiotherapy and exercise training are the most important to clear tracheobronchial secretion and to preserve airway patency.
4. Adequate oxygenation: The dangers of oxygen therapy in chronic respiratory failure should be borne in mind. The risk of respiratory depression is always there and sensible precautions should be taken. Humidification of inspired gases may help expectoration.
5. Management of such respiratory cripple patients should aim to maximize the pulmonary function, to reduce the frequency of acute attacks and to treat complications of hypoxemia.

Management of Acute Exacerbations

1. Adequate oxygenation, and IPPV
2. Bronchodilator therapy
3. Antibiotics
4. Chest percussion and postural drainage
5. Corticosteroids
6. Mucolytic agents
7. Tracheobronchial toilet and care
8. Other supportive measures
9. Adequate nutrition.

Pulmonary Embolism

Pulmonary embolism may be defined as the partial or complete obstruction of the pulmonary arterial circulation by some substances such as thrombus, fat, air, amniotic fluid, etc. migrated to the lung from elsewhere in the body. Massive pulmonary embolism often results in sudden cardiovascular collapse and death. It is mostly due to acute reduction of cardiac output, acute right ventricular failure and disturbance of pulmonary perfusion and ventilation.

Predisposing Factors

1. Deep vein thrombosis
2. Recent fracture and/or leg injury
3. Prolonged immobilization
4. Major abdominal or orthopedic surgery
5. Varicose veins
6. Pregnancy and patients with oral contraceptives
7. Cardiac failure and atrial fibrillation
8. Smoking, obesity, and polycythemia vera.

Main Types of Emboli

1. **Thromboembolus**: It is mostly due to venous stasis of blood, hypercoagulability of blood and abnormalities or damage of vessel wall. Prolonged immobilization or bed rest may be a factor. Spontaneous dislodgement can occur.
2. **Fat embolus**: It is mostly due to fracture of long bones, sternal slitting operation, trauma or injury to subcutaneous fat, etc. It may occur 12–24 hours after injury.
3. **Air embolus**: Air usually enters the circulation through the venous system. A 100 ml of air may be fatal. Infusion of air or other gas under pressure into the vein in IV lines may cause air embolism. Other causes include pulmonary artery balloon rupture, tubal insufflation, hemodialysis, chest trauma, neck surgery, rapid decompression, and so on.

4. **Miscellaneous**: Amniotic fluid, sheared catheter tip, infected tissue or tissue fragment, etc. may cause embolism.
5. **Predisposing factors regarding venous thrombosis and pulmonary embolism**: Prolonged bed rest, trauma, surgery, obesity, pregnancy, congestive cardiac failure, oral contraceptives, and general immobility.

Pathophysiology

1. These emboli may travel through both the venous and arterial system. It is said that right lung is involved more than left and lower lobes more than the upper lobes. Small emboli less than 4 mm in diameter rarely become problematic, but larger emboli may cause serious problems.
2. Pulmonary embolism increases pulmonary dead space and there is mismatched ventilation—Perfusion.
3. Loss of surfactant also occurs and it causes alveolar collapse, atelectasis, shunting of blood, and hypoxemia.
4. Pulmonary artery hypertension occurs mostly due to mechanical obstruction in pulmonary vascular bed. Right ventricular failure is common.
5. Bronchoconstriction and bronchospasm can also occur.
6. The dual blood supply of lungs (pulmonary and bronchial arterial systems) and good collateral circulation may be beneficial in such patients.

Clinical Manifestations

1. Sudden onset of acute dyspnea, confusion, agitation, and loss of consciousness.
2. Pleuritic chest pain.
3. Hemoptysis.

4. Tachypnea, nonproductive cough, and hypoxemia.
5. Tachycardia, profuse perspiration, cyanosis, hypotension, and atrial arrhythmias.
6. Wheezing and moist sound over lung fields.
7. Acute right ventricular failure. There may be elevation of jugular venous pressure and gallop rhythm at left sternal angle.
8. Acute drop in cardiac output.
9. Cardiopulmonary arrest.
10. In amniotic fluid embolism squames may be found on microscopic examination of sputum.
11. In air embolism in the right ventricle there may be churning sound on auscultation.
12. In fat embolism, petechial rash may be seen on chest, shoulders, and axillae. DIC, thrombocytopenia, bleeding, fat globules in urine, sputum and retinal vessels, hypoxemia, confusion, coma, convulsion, fever, and ARDS.
13. Features of minor pulmonary embolism include chest pain, pleural friction rub with signs of consolidation or crepitations, cough, and hemoptysis.

Investigations

1. **Chest X-ray**: Usually normal, pleural effusion, pulmonary edema, and atelectasis.
2. **Pulmonary angiogram**: It gives definitive diagnosis. Hemodynamic studies can be performed while catheters are in situ.
3. **Electrocardiogram**: Acute cor pulmonale and right heart strain.
4. **Arterial blood gas analysis**: Decreased PaO_2, increased $PaCO_2$, and respiratory acidosis. Increased A/a gradient even with an FiO_2 of 100%.
5. **Serum lipase**: Increased in fat embolism.

6. Serum lactate dehydrogenase: Increased.
7. Lung scan: Low uptake of ^{131}I with normal chest X-ray is very suggestive of embolism.
8. Total blood count.
9. Coagulation studies.
10. Hemodynamic monitoring: Sudden increase in pulmonary artery pressure.
11. Examination of urine.
12. Examination of sputum.

Management

1. **Cardiopulmonary support**
   a. IV central line
   b. Volume expanders to improve cardiac output
   c. Oxygen therapy
   d. Mechanical ventilation: IPPV
   e. External cardiac massage and IPPV in cases of sudden cardiac arrest
   f. Inotropic drugs: Isoprenaline and dopamine
   g. Reversal of metabolic acidosis: 8.4% sodium bicarbonate
   h. Heparin
   i. Diuretics
   j. Steroids.
2. **Definitive treatment**
   a. *Embolectomy*: Pulmonary artery embolectomy is only indicated in cases of massive emboli. Cardiopulmonary bypass should be used.
   b. *Anticoagulants*: Heparin decreases clotting ability of blood and thus prevents thromboembolus.
   c. *Systemic fibrinolytic therapy*: Streptokinase or urokinase is used to hasten resolution of emboli. It is best effective when the clot is less than 3 days old. But it may cause uncontrolled bleeding and cardiac

arrhythmias. The therapy needs laboratory control with thrombin clotting time. Streptokinase therapy is contraindicated in cases of internal bleeding and history of cerebrovascular accident, hemorrhagic diathesis and severe hypertension. Relative contraindications may include asthma, allergic patients, pregnancy, elderly patients, inflammatory bowel disease, etc.

3. In cases with air embolus, the patient should be placed on left side in head down position, so air will float into the right atrium.
   - Aspiration of the air from right atrium can be done through a central line inserted into right atrium.
4. **Treatment of acute massive pulmonary embolism**:
   a. External cardiac massage
   b. Oxygen therapy
   c. Heparin IV
   d. Treatment of acidosis
   e. Definitive measures:
      i. Anticoagulants
      ii. Fibrinolytic therapy
      iii. Surgical intervention.
5. **Prophylaxis**:
   a. *Anticoagulant therapy*: Heparin may be indicated.
   b. Inferior vena cava interruption may be indicated in some cases to prevent further emboli. It is usually done with a transvenous umbrella filter or with surgically placed clip on the vessel. It is indicated in cases of recurrent emboli, septic emboli, critically ill patients, and when heparin therapy is not possible.

Pneumothorax

Pneumothorax is usually defined as the presence of air in the pleural space from an injury of chest wall or more commonly from an air leak of the lung. There may be either connection of the atmosphere to the pleural space or rupture of alveolus into the pleural cavity.

Causes

1. **Chest injury**: Penetrating chest injury, fracture of ribs, and lung laceration.
2. Spontaneous rupture of emphysematous bullae.
3. IPPV with PEEP.
4. Rupture of esophagus, damage to a bronchus or trachea.
5. Regional block of nerves or surgery in close proximity to pleural cavity.
6. Barotrauma.
7. During laparoscopy (due to CO_2 insufflation).
8. Following diagnostic procedures like bronchoscopy, esophagoscopy, pleurocentesis, lung biopsy, liver biopsy, and following CVP line placement.

Types of Pneumothorax

1. **Simple pneumothorax**: Minor leak of air causing mild degree of lung collapse. Leak usually seals and air is absorbed. No chest tube drainage is needed.
2. **Open pneumothorax**: Leak has a free communication with the atmosphere either through a bronchopleural fistula or a wound in chest wall.
3. **Closed pneumothorax**: Air accumulates in closed intrathoracic cavity and there is no communication with the atmosphere. A valve system at the leak can occur when the air can enter, but cannot escape leading to tension pneumothorax. This causes shifting of mediastinum and displacement of major vessels. Venous return to the heart decreases and cardiovascular collapse results. It can cause sudden death.

Clinical Features

1. History of chronic bronchitis, asthma, chronic obstructive airway disease, emphysema, lung cyst, and bronchopleural fistula.
2. History of chest injury and fracture of ribs.
3. Chest pain, agitation, apprehension, shortness of breath, cough, and shoulder pain.
4. In severe cases nausea/vomiting, syncope, and shock.
5. **Closed pneumothorax**:
   a. Dyspnea, tachypnea, and cyanosis.
   b. Diminished breath sounds over the affected site.
   c. Hypoxemia.
6. **Open pneumothorax**: Added findings are:
   a. Open injury at affected site.
   b. Sucking sound on inspiration at affected site.
   c. Subcutaneous emphysema.
7. **Tension pneumothorax**: Added findings are:
   a. Asymetric movement of chest.
   b. Deviation of trachea to unaffected side.
   c. Reduced venous return.
   d. Tachycardia, low blood pressure, and shock.
   e. Heart sounds muffled.

Diagnosis

1. **Chest X-ray**: It is most helpful to detect pneumothorax. In tension pneumothorax there are features of mediastinal shift, tracheal deviation and area of air without lung markings.
   - An apical pneumothorax may show a cap of air and it should be carefully observed. It should also be determined whether there is fluid indicating hemopneumothorax. Pre-existing lung disease can also be ascertained.

2. **Hemodynamic monitoring**: Cardiac output, pulmonary wedge pressure, and central venous pressure may need monitoring.
3. **Pulmonary function tests**: Decreased lung function.
4. CT scan of chest.

Management

Prevention

1. Identification of patients at risk of pneumothorax.
2. Nitrous oxide should be avoided in such cases.
3. CVP lines should be placed carefully.
4. Ventilation with high pressure should be avoided. Patients with long-term IPPV need regular chest X-ray to exclude pneumothorax.
5. Regional block or surgery very close to pleural cavity needs extra caution.

Treatment

1. **Closed pneumothorax**:
   a. If pneumothorax is small and less than 20%, usually no treatment is needed.
   b. Re-expansion of the lung should be promoted.
      - Insertion of an intercostal catheter attached to an underwater seal. It is usually done under local anesthesia into the axillary area. Escape of the air should be slow, otherwise sudden changes in intrapleural pressure can cause acute pulmonary edema and rapid mediastinal shift may cause problems. Serial X-rays of chest will assess the re-expansion of the lungs. Frequent assessment of breath sounds is also needed.
   c. Chest drainage should be assessed.
   d. Serial arterial blood gas analysis and chest X-ray are always helpful.

2. **Open pneumothorax**:
   a. This is a more serious condition. In addition to the measures for simple closed pneumothorax, the wound needs careful attention. Sterile occlusive dressing over the wound is always helpful. But if a tension pneumothorax develops, the wound will be uncovered and insertion of chest tube is indicated. Tension pneumothorax can be diagnosed by tracheal deviation, jugular vein distension and acute respiratory distress.
3. **Tension pneumothorax**:
   a. Early recognition is most important.
   b. In acute emergency situation, needle decompression using a 14–16 gauge needle at the second intercostal space, midclavicular line on affected side is most indicated.
   c. Insertion of chest tube with underwater drain must be done once the emergency is over.
4. **Other supportive measures**:
   a. Adequate oxygenation: Airway clearance
   b. Prevention of infection: Antibiotics
   c. Pain relief: Analgesics
   d. Monitoring of vital signs.
5. **Definitive surgical intervention may be needed in cases of**:
   a. Bilateral pneumothorax
   b. If pneumothorax remains open
   c. Recurrent pneumothorax.

Complications

1. Hypoxemia
2. Hypotension and shock
3. Cardiac arrhythmias
4. Venous or arterial gas embolism
5. Cardiac arrest.

Aspiration Pneumonitis

Aspiration pneumonitis is characterized by destruction of surfactant producing cells resulting atelectasis and damage to pulmonary capillary endothelium causing intravascular fluid leaks into the lungs due to the aspiration of gastric fluid into the lungs.

Predisposing Factors

1. Common in children, elderly patients, obstetric pateints, patients with full stomach and vomiting prone type of patients.
2. Patients with impaired laryngeal reflexes, altered level of consciousness, anesthesia of larynx and pharynx, muscle weakness or paralysis, acute intoxication of alcohol.
3. Patients with incompetent gastroesophageal junction: Hiatus hernia, previous esophageal surgery.
4. Passive regurgitation and active vomiting.

Pathophysiology

1. It is mostly due to massive aspiration of gastric contents. Severity of lung damage depends on pH, volume, and distribution of the aspirated material into the lungs. Aspiration of food matters may also be a factor. Aspiration of hypertonic solutions, irritating food matters, infected materials, and foreign bodies may also be responsible.
2. Initially reflex airways closure, alteration of surfactant, interstitial and alveolar edema, obstruction of smaller airways, intrapulmonary shunts, increased lung water, and loss of pulmonary compliance. All these lead to hypoxemia.

3. Highly acidic material causes loss of alveolar capillary permeability, severe inflammation, edema, hemorrhage and necrosis of airways and lung parenchyma. Excessive lung damage causes loss of intravascular volume, hypotension, and shock.
4. Critical pH value of the aspirate is 2.5; above pH 2.5, the response is mostly similar to that of distilled water; pH below 1.5, pulmonary damage is maximum.
5. Volume of the aspirate is also a factor. The critical volume of the aspirate is 25 ml. The volume more than 25 ml causes much damage.
6. Infected aspirate material causes infection and lung abscess, empyema or necrotising bacterial pneumonia can occur.

Clinical Features

1. It will depend on the character and type of aspirate, volume, pH, and distribution of the aspirate in lung parenchyma.
2. Particulate aspirate may cause airway obstruction, severe hypoxemia, and even cardiorespiratory arrest.
3. Small infected material may not show any symptoms initially; but, later on, there may be features of lung abscess and lobar pneumonia.
4. Aspiration of gastric contents with a pH less than 2.5 and volume more than 25 ml cause chemical burns and aspiration pneumonitis. There may be bronchospasm, dyspnea, tachypnea, cyanosis, hypotension, wheezing, and crepitations. Arterial hypoxemia is the main feature.
5. Due to obstruction and atelectasis, there is shunting of arteriolar blood with a widening of alveolar arterial oxygen gradient. Noncardiogenic pulmonary edema, adult respiratory distress syndrome will result. There

are decreased pulmonary compliance, ventilation perfusion defect and significant intrapulmonary shunting.

Investigations

1. **Chest X-ray**: May remain normal for first 6–12 hours after aspiration. Later, patchy pneumonitis with irregular soft mottled densities in the peripheral lung fields. Atelectasis may also be there.
2. **Arterial blood gas analysis**: Hypoxemia, hypercarbia, and acidosis.
3. Total blood count.

Management

Prophylactic Measures

1. Aspiration pneumonitis is most common at the time of induction of anesthesia. So adequate preparation is essential. Preanesthetic fasting for 4–6 hours is needed. General anesthesia should be avoided in patients with full stomach.
2. Laryngeal competence may be decreased for 4–8 hours following extubation. Thus, adequate care is needed during early postoperative period.
3. Patients at risk should be identified and adequate precautions should be taken. Patients with gravid uterus, intra-abdominal injury, intestinal obstruction, etc. may have gastric emptying time much longer.
4. Proper pharyngeal pack is needed following endotracheal intubation. Cuff must be efficient.
5. Nasogastric suction at frequent intervals is often helpful.
6. Some drugs like anticholinergic drugs, ganglion blocking drugs, opioids, thiopentone, tricyclic

antidepressant drugs, etc. may reduce the lower esophageal sphincter pressure and increase the tendency to gastroesophageal reflux.
7. Position of the patient is important. The patient should be placed in a position in which the tracheobronchial tree is at downward angle.
8. *Neutralization of gastric contents may be tried by some drugs*:
   a. Magnesium trisilicate gel.
   b. Sodium citrate.
   c. *H_2 receptor blocking agents*: Cimetidine, ranitidine, famotidine, etc.
   d. Metoclopramide is helpful in reducing gastric volume as it shortens the gastric emptying time. It also reduces the incidence and severity of vomiting.
9. Vomiting-prone type of patients should also be identified. Antiemetic drugs like prochlorperazine, ondansetron, etc. may be given.

Treatment

Massive aspiration of gastric contents should be detected early and managed immediately.
1. Head down tilt.
2. Tracheobronchial toilet. Lavage and suction may be needed to remove particulate material.
3. Bronchoscopic suction.
4. *Adequate oxygenation*: IPPV with 100% oxygen and PEEP.
5. Ventilatory support: PEEP or continuous positive airway pressure may be helpful to maintain adequate oxygenation and normalize blood gas defects.
6. Hydrocortisone instillation in tracheobronchial tree is often helpful.
7. Bronchodilator drugs to relieve bronchospasm. Albuterol by metered dose inhaler may be effective.

8. Steroids IV may be beneficial.
9. Broad-spectrum antibiotics.
10. *IV infusion of fluids*: Overinfusion should be avoided.
11. Diuretics should be used with sensible precautions.
12. Monitoring of intrapulmonary shunt, wedge pressure and cardiac output is essential in critically ill patients. Pulmonary artery wedge pressure monitoring is often helpful.
13. Monitoring of vital signs and blood gas analysis should be routine.
14. Frequent lung assessment is also needed.

Complications

1. Pneumonia
2. Sepsis
3. Adult respiratory distress syndrome.

Upper Airway Obstruction

Upper airway obstruction is a serious life-threatening condition that requires rapid evaluation of the patient and simultaneous therapy to provide adequate oxygenation and ventilation. Prompt recognition of the patient's condition is the most important for planning the patient care without wasting time.

Common Causes

Laryngospasm, foreign bodies, trauma, tumors, epiglottitis, Ludwig's angina, odontogenic abscess, peritonsillar abscess, tonsillar enlargement, laryngotracheitis, diphtheria, burns, inhalation injury, foreign body aspiration, hemorrhage into the neck, intraoral hemorrhage, damage to recurrent laryngeal nerves, collapsing trachea, etc.

Clinical Features

Inability to phonate either partial or complete, rocking movement of the chest with inadequate air exchange, tracheal tug, flaring of nostrils, increased respiratory movements, cyanosis, inspiratory stridor.

Arterial blood gas analysis is helpful in diagnosing hypoventilation.

Note

1. Expiratory wheezing is common in small lower airway obstruction.
2. Noisy auditory signs are commonly associated with partial airway obstruction.

Step by step guidelines for management of upper airway obstruction:

1. Adequate airway should be either established or maintained. Head tilt and chin lift should be tried.
2. Mask ventilation may be needed.
3. Endotracheal intubation should be done only if necessary.
4. If mask ventilation and intubation fail, transtracheal oxygenation is helpful. Transtracheal ventilation should not be done.
5. Tracheostomy in extreme cases.
6. Associated cardiovascular instability should be treated when ventilation is established.
7. Lastly the exact cause of hypoventilation should be diagnosed and additional management is based on etiology.

Note

1. The expert help experienced in difficult airways may be needed.

2. Tracheostomy set and intubation equipment may be needed. Indirect laryngoscopy or fiber optic nasopharyngolaryngoscope should always to cautious.
3. Close monitoring of vital signs is essential.
4. General supportive care.

Airway Burn

Airway burn can occur due to thermal or chemical injury to mucosa of airway extending from nose/mouth to alveoli. Thermal injury is usually due to inhalation of hot gases/ vapors, or directly from fire and/or smoke. During laser surgery the endotracheal tube can ignite and cause airway burn. Faulty inspired gas heater or humidifier may also be responsible.

Clinical Features

All patients in closed space fires usually suffer from inhalation injury particularly in burns of face and neck, involvement of proximal airway can cause rapid edema and obstruction. Soft tissue swelling of the face, oropharynx, glottis, and trachea is common. There may be carbon deposits in the nasopharynx and oropharynx, expectorated carbonaceous sputum, wheezing, respiratory insufficiency, hypoxemia and increased carbon monoxide level in blood. There are decreased arterial PO_2 and O_2 saturation, decreased pulmonary compliance, pulmonary edema, bronchospasm and eventually leading to adult respiratory distress syndrome (ARDS). Management should include administration of 100% oxygen, early intubation and mechanical ventilation and general supportive care.

In cases of laser-ignited endotracheal fire:
1. Ignition or burning of the tube may be seen

2. Smell of burning, smoke, and flames
3. Fire can extend to breathing circuit.

Management

1. Patient should be disconnected from the breathing circuit. Flow of oxygen should be stopped through the tube.
2. The damaged tube should be taken out.
3. Mask ventilation with 100% oxygen.
4. Reintubation is tried, if possible.
5. Mechanical ventilation with PEEP.
6. Steroids.
7. Supportive care.
8. **Prevention**:
   a. Use of protected endotracheal tube (laser-proof).
   b. Cuff should be filled with colored water or saline.
   c. Avoid nitrous oxide.
   d. Careful monitoring.

In cases with overheated gases/vapors:

i. Breathing circuit becomes hot.
ii. High rise of patient's body temperature.
iii. High temperature alarm sounds may be heard.
iv. Management should include:
   a. Removal of heater/humidifier from the circuit.
   b. Careful evaluation.
   c. Maintain adequate oxygenation.
   d. Steroids.
   e. Fiber optic bronchoscopy, when the condition is stable.
   f. General supportive care.

Flail Chest

Flail chest can result from direct high energy force over the chest wall. Broken ribs are very painful and cause splinting with ventilation-perfusion mismatching. Flail segment commonly involves anterior or lateral rib fractures, posterior rib fractures usually do not cause flail segment due to good stability provided by muscles. Usually two or more ribs are fractured in two or more sites. Paradoxical motion of that chest wall segment is often present. Flail segments can also cause inefficient ventilation and atelectasis.

Blunt force of injury mostly cause pulmonary contusion. In such cases hemoptysis and atelectasis can occur. Pneumothorax and hydrothorax can also result. Associated other injuries particularly abdominal injuries may be present. Diagnosis is confirmed by chest X-ray.

Management

1. Assess the patient very carefully. There may be shock and respiratory distress. Labored breathing, increased respiratory rate, low oxygen saturation and $PaO_2 < 60$ min Hg indicate respiratory insufficiency.
2. In presence of shock and/or respiratory insufficiency endotracheal intubation and IPPV with 100% O_2 are indicated. In patients with positive pressure ventilation paradoxical movement of chest wall segment may not be seen. Continuous positive airway pressure (CPAP) is often helpful.
3. **Pain control is most important**:
   a. Systemic opioids by continuous infusion.
   b. Patient controlled anesthesia.
   c. Regional anesthesia: Epidural block.
   d. Intercostal nerve blocks.
4. Close monitoring particularly pulse oximetry and continuous end-tidal CO_2 is needed.
5. General supportive care provides pulmonary hygiene and physiotherapy (cough-deep breathing).

Chapter 2

Cardiovascular Disorders

Acute Myocardial Infarction

Acute myocardial infarction is characterized by the damage of myocardial tissue mostly due to occlusive coronary disease resulting in permanent loss of contractility to that part of myocardial muscle. It is myocardial cell death due to inadequate cellular perfusion.

Angina pectoris is described as chest discomfort mostly due to myocardial ischemia. There is a sensation of retrosternal dullness, constrictive or heaviness which may radiate to the arms, neck, and jaw. It may be precipitated by exertion, exercise, emotion, and some environmental circumstances which increase the myocardial oxygen demand or cause coronary artery spasm. Acute myocardial infarction may not always be associated with angina. It is said that 10%–15% cases of acute myocardial infarction are silent.

Angina pectoris occuring with less than normal activity or lasting for more prolonged period than before is taken as characteristic of unstable angina and may march towards acute myocardial infarction. Angina pectoris is said to be stable when there is no change in the precipitating factors, frequency and duration of pain for at least 60 days. It is easily controlled with rest or nitroglycerin.

Risk Factors

1. Male sex: Patients with angina pectoris.
2. Elderly subjects.
3. Hypercholesterolemia.
4. Hypertension: Patients with aortic or mitral stenosis.
5. Smoking.
6. Metabolic diseases; diabetes mellitus and obesity.
7. Sedentary lifestyle.
8. Family history.
9. Psychosocial characteristics: Aggressiveness, competitiveness, etc.

Causes

1. Coronary atherosclerosis: Acute occlusion of coronary artery.
2. Coronary thrombosis.
3. Coronary spasm.
4. Profound shock and hypotension. Inadequate coronary perfusion.
5. Cardiac trauma.

Diagnosis

Clinical Features

1. *Chest pain*: Retrosternal, may or may not, radiate to the arms, shoulders or neck. Dull, aching, deep strangling, tightness, squeezing, crushing, pressure or heaviness. Dyspnea: It may last longer than 15 – 30 minutes. Rest and nitroglycerine are mostly ineffective. Relieved by morphine. Patients with peripheral neuropathy (diabetic) or altered sensorium may mask the pain sensation.
2. Weakness and fatigue.

3. Nausea/vomiting.
4. Rise of body temperature.
5. Decreased level of consciousness.
6. Labile blood pressure may be increased or decreased. Tachycardia/bradycardia.

Investigations

1. **Electrocardiogram**: ST depression and/or T-wave inversion may indicate ischemia. ST segment elevation is found in acute myocardial infarction or coronary spasm. Q-waves indicate infarction.
2. **Cardiac monitoring**: Sinus bradycardia, atrioventricular blocks, atrial fibrillation or flutter, premature ventricular beats. Ventricular tachycardia and ventricular fibrillation.
3. Echocardiography.
4. **Hemodynamic monitoring**: Increased pulmonary artery pressure, pulmonary capillary wedge pressure. Decreased cardiac output.
5. **Radioisotope imaging**: Thalium scan and radionuclide angiocardiography.
6. **Angiography**: Coronary angiography is the definitive test for coronary artery disease.
7. Cardiac catheterization.
8. Magnetic resonance imaging.
9. **Laboratory tests**:
    a. *Cardiac enzymes*: Increased creatine kinase.
    b. Transient increases in plasma concentration of myocardial enzymes, CK-MB increases during first 4–12 hours in more than 50% cases.
    c. Aspertate aminotransferase (SGOT) increases.
    d. LDH increases.
    e. WBC count increases within 48 hours.
    f. ESR increases.

10. **Chest X-ray**: Pulmonary congestion, and left ventricular failure.

Management

1. Myocardial oxygen consumption should be reduced:
   a. Complete bed rest.
   b. Drugs like nitrates, opioids, β-blockers, calcium channel blockers, and sedatives.
2. Myocardial oxygen supply should be increased:
   a. Adequate oxygenation
   b. Some medications need consideration:
      i. Thrombolytics
      ii. Aspirin
      iii. Anticoagulants.
3. Artificial cardiac pacemaker. If cardiac arrest occurs, CPR should be started immediately.
4. Emergency coronary arteriography and percutaneous transluminal coronary angioplasty.
5. Further cardiovascular damage should be assessed and prevention should be tried:
   a. Monitor vital signs.
   b. Continuous ECG monitoring.
   c. Continuous cardiac monitoring.
   d. IV line should be established and IV infusion is needed. Insertion of central line may be indicated. Optimise circulating fluid volume.
   e. Some medications may be needed:
      i. Antiarrhythmic drugs
      ii. Nitrates
      iii. Inotropic drugs.
6. Nutritional care.
7. Bowel care: Stool softeners and mild laxatives.
8. Rehabilitation.

Drug Therapy

1. **Thrombolytic agents**: Tissue plasminogen activator, streptokinase. It helps to dissolve blood clots obstructing coronary arteries. It should be given within 6 hours of attack. There is a risk of intracranial hemorrhage. Reocclusion may occur in some cases.
2. **Nitrates**: Nitroglycerin reduces cardiac workload by peripheral vasodilation. It dilates coronary arteries and thus reduces angina. However, it can cause headache, hypotension, poor tissue perfusion, and reflex tachycardia.
3. **Opioids**: It relieves pain, anxiety and reduces cardiac workload, but it can cause hypotension and bradycardia.
4. **Antiarrhythmic drugs**: Lignocaine reduces the incidence of cardiac arrhythmias.
5. β-blockers like metoprolol reduces myocardial oxygen consumption by decreased heart rate, blood pressure and cardiac output. But it may exacerbate heart failure and shock. Esmolol, labetolol or propranolol should be used with caution.
6. **Inotropic drugs**: Dobutamine may augment coronary circulation by increasing cardiac output and decreasing pulmonary artery pressure and systemic vascular resistance.

Complications of Acute Myocardial Infarction

1. Cardiac dysrhythmia and conduction defects
2. Pericarditis and pericardial effusion
3. Left ventricular thrombus
4. Congestive cardiac failure
5. Cardiogenic shock and hemodynamic instability
6. Ventricular septal rupture

7. Acute mitral regurgitation.
8. Ventricular aneurysm and pulmonary embolism.
9. Cardiac rupture.
10. Cardiorespiratory arrest. Cardiac asystole.

General Considerations

1. Patients at risk should be identified and some preventive measures may be adopted.
2. Patient and family education regarding the disease is essential.
3. Risk factors and conditions known to precipitate symptoms should be avoided as far as practicable.
4. Cessation of smoking and alcohol.
5. Hypertension, diabetes mellitus, hyperlipidemia should be controlled.
6. Weight reduction, proper exercise, and removal of stressful physical and mental stimuli are always helpful.
7. Avoid elective anesthesia and surgery in cases with unstable angina or with past history of myocardial infarction in the previous 6 months. Hemodynamics and hematocrit should be optimized during anesthesia and surgery.

Congestive Cardiac Failure

Congestive cardiac failure implies the inability of the heart to pump an adequate amount of blood to the vital organs of the body to meet the metabolic needs.

Causes

1. **Cardiac valve abnormality**:
   a. Causing abnormal pressure loads:

i. Aorta stenosis.
   ii. Pulmonary stenosis.
 b. Causing abnormal filling of ventricles:
   i. Mitral stenosis.
   ii. Tricuspid stenosis.
2. **Abnormal myocardial contractility**:
   a. Cardiomyopathy
   b. Secondary to ischemic heart disease
   c. Myocarditis
   d. Myocardial infarction.
3. **Abnormal volume load**:
   a. Aortic regurgitation
   b. Mitral regurgitation
   c. Pulmonary regurgitation
   d. Tricuspid regurgitation.
4. **Systemic hypertension**.
5. **Pulmonary hypertension**.

Congestive heart failure is usually described as right-sided failure or left-sided failure. As the cardiopulmonary system is a closed one, the effects of one-sided cardiac failure will ultimately affect the other side.

Left-sided heart failure may occur when the left ventricle fails to pump oxygenated blood from pulmonary circulation to the systemic circulation. This is mostly due to systemic hypertension, coronary artery disease, valvular heart disease (aortic stenosis) and cardiomyopathy.

Right heart failure may be secondary to left heart failure, pulmonary hypertension, pulmonary stenosis and so on. Hypoxia in such cases increases pulmonary vascular resistance and eventually right ventricular failure.

Clinical Manifestations

1. **Left-sided heart failure**: Fatigue, anxiety, shortness of breath, paroxysmal nocturnal dyspnea, exertional

dyspnea, orthopnea, confusion, pulmonary congestion, rales, coughing, pleural effusion, tachycardia, peripheral edema, oliguria, acute pulmonary edema, and so on.
2. **Right-sided heart failure**: Heaviness of legs, systemic venous congestion, hepatomegaly, ascites, dependent and pitting peripheral edema, tachycardia, jugular vein distension, weight gain, etc.

Acute attack is most common in acute infection and in chronic obstructive airway disease. Biventricular failure is always associated with fluid overload and hypoalbuminemia.

Investigations

1. **Chest X-ray**: Pulmonary congestion, fluid accumulation in lung fields, ventricular hypertrophy, and cardiomegaly.
2. **Electrocardiogram**: Infarction, ischemia, arrhythmias, and ventricular enlargement.
3. **Echocardiogram**: Dilation of cardiac chambers, dysfunction of valves, and ventricular hypertrophy.
4. Radionuclide angiocardiography.
5. **Hemodynamic monitoring**: Increased central venous pressure, pulmonary capillary wedge pressure, and right atrial pressure.
6. **Cardiac catheterization**: Increased pressure within the heart chambers and the pulmonary vascular system.
7. **Laboratory findings**:
   a. Arterial blood gas analysis: Decreased PaO_2, increased $PaCO_2$, and decreased pH.
   b. Cardiac enzymes and isoenzymes increased.
   c. Serum lactate increased.
   d. Liver function tests impaired.
   e. Blood biochemistry: Urea and creatinine increased.
   f. Total blood count.

Management

1. Adequate oxygenation either through nasal cannula or through endotracheal tube. Mechanical ventilation may be needed—IPPV.
2. Oxygen saturation should be continuously monitored. Pulse oximeter should be applied. Serial arterial blood gas analysis is needed.
3. The exact cause of cardiac failure should be ascertained. Workload on the heart should be decreased.
4. Maintain bed rest. Slight head up-tilt, if the patient tolerates.
5. IV line should be established. Fluid should be given cautiously. Overhydration is always harmful.
6. Cardiac monitoring, monitoring of central venous pressure, and pulmonary artery pressure is always helpful. Monitoring of vital signs is essential.
7. Ascites or pleural effusion may cause cardiorespiratory embarassment and may need tapping with usual precautions.
8. Hypoxia, hypotension, and unnecessary increase in the workload on the heart should be avoided.
9. Drug therapy is most important.
   a. Digitalis is most commonly used as positive inotropic drug. It is orally effective and excreted mostly by the kidneys. Several preparations are available. It should be used cautiously as digitalis toxicity can occur.
   b. Dopamine, dobutamine (β-agonists): It increases cardiac muscle contractility and subsequently cardiac output. It can cause arrhythmias, tachycardia and peripheral vasoconstriction. It is better to monitor the effects of β-agonists on cardiac output and cardiac filling pressures using pulmonary artery catheter.

c. Diuretics: Frusemide—It decreases fluid volume efficiently. Prolonged use can cause electrolyte imbalance. Chronic oral administration of loop diuretics can cause hypovolemia, orthostatic hypotension, and hypokalemia.

d. Vasodilators: Nitroglycerin, sodium nitroprusside. The aim should be to optimize cardiac output by manipulating the peripheral circulation with vasodilators. Vasodilators increase cardiac output by decreasing impedence to the forward ejection of left ventricular stroke volume. But it may cause severe hypotension and thus invasive monitoring like arterial and pulmonary artery catheter is always beneficial.

Captopril interrupts the conversion of angiotensin I to angiotensin II, vasodilates arteriolar and venous system, decreases the level of circulating catecholamines and decreases myocardial oxygen demand. But it can increase serum potassium levels and cause hypotension. It should not be used in patients suffering from renal disease or diabetes mellitus.

e. Opioid analgesics: It decreases arterial blood pressure and systemic vascular resistance, vasodilates and relieves anxiety and pain. But it can cause respiratory depression and hypotension.

10. General measures:
   a. Careful monitoring of respiratory status, cardiovascular status and hemodynamics is essential.
   b. Monitor fluid and electrolyte status: Maintain intake output balance. Overloading the circulation may worsen the cardiac failure and precipitate pulmonary edema. Restrict water and sodium intake. Body weight should be taken at same time

on same scale.
  c. Life-threatening emergencies may occur. It should be prevented and managed accordingly:
     i. Rupture of papillary muscle.
     ii. Rupture of interventricular septum.
     iii. Pulmonary edema.
  d. Some precipitating factors may worsen the condition and adquate precautions should be taken against them:
     i. Dietary or parenteral sodium load, fluid overload.
     ii. Sodium-retaining drugs like corticosteroids.
     iii. Cardiac depressant drugs: β-blockers and calcium channel blockers.
     iv. Stress: Emotional, physical, and environmental.
     v. Increased metabolic demand: Fever, anemia, hyperthyroidism, obesity, and pregnancy.
     vi. Poor pulmonary/renal function.
     vii. Arrhythmias.
     viii. Pulmonary emboli, coarctation, and A-V fistula.
     ix. Drug interactions.

Acute Pulmonary Edema

Acute pulmonary edema is characterized by the accumulation of fluid in the pulmonary interstitial or alveolar spaces. It may be of two types, cardiogenic and noncardiogenic pulmonary edema. Noncardiogenic pulmonary edema, better known as adult respiratory distress syndrome (ARDS) is already discussed in this volume. Here cardiogenic edema is being dealt in some details.

Cardiogenic pulmonary edema results when the pulmonary capillary pressure exceeds the pressures, serum osmotic pressure and interstitial hydrostatic pressure, which keep fluid in the intravascular space. Increased pulmonary capillary pressure causes accumulation of fluid in the pulmonary interstitial space and then in alveolar spaces. This is mostly due to cardiac dysfunction like left ventricular failure, obstruction to transmitral blood flow as in mitral stenosis, atrial myxoma and veno-occlusive disease.

- Patients at risk for pulmonary edema:
    1. *Increased pulmonary capillary wedge pressure*:
        a. Overloading the circulation.
        b. Acute myocardial infarction.
        c. Decompensating chronic heart failure.
        d. Mitral valve diseases and mitral stenosis.
        e. Aortic stenosis.
        f. Severe hypertension.
        g. Massive pulmonary embolism.
        h. Central nervous system diseases and neurologic diseases.
    2. *Decreased lymphatic drainage of normal alveolar fluid*: (Inadequate lymphatic clearance)
        a. Pneumonia.
        b. Pulmonary injury.
        c. Microemboli.
        d. Increased central venous pressure from any case.
- Factors that may worsen cardiogenic pulmonary edema:
    1. Hypoalbuminemia decreases the serum osmotic pressure and reduces the pulmonary capillary pressure at which transudation occurs.
    2. Decreased pulmonary interstitial pressure as in rapid removal of huge pleural fluid.
    3. Primary alveolar capillary membrane damage as in cases of prolonged hypotension and exposure to toxins.

4. Primary lymphatic dysfunction.
5. Neurologic diseases, and narcotic overdose.
6. Anxiety, catecholamine release, etc.

Pathophysiology

1. Acute pulmonary edema diminishes the effective lung tissue essential for gas exchange. It also impairs the diffusion between the alveoli and capillary. Increased capillary permeability (as in shock and sepsis), increased hydrostatic pressure in the capillaries (as in fluid overload and congestive heart failure) and decreased plasma osmotic pressure (as in hypoalbuminemia) are main factors for causing pulmonary edema.
2. Increased left atrial and left ventricular pressure may cause acute pulmonary edema. It may have four stages. Initially, lung parenchyma swells and lymphatics are unable to absorb excess fluid. Then, there is excess fluid in alveoli resulting hypoxemia, tachypnea, increased venous return to heart and increased blood volume within the pulmonary capillary bed. Later, the surfactant activity is impaired, atelectasis occurs and ultimately there are tissue hypoxia, hypoventilation, and acidosis.
3. Acute myocardial ischemia or infarction.
4. Neurogenic following major head injury.

Clinical Features

1. History of recent acute myocardial infarction.
2. Anxiety, dyspnea, orthopnea, air hunger, and restlessness.
3. Coughing and blood-tinged frothy sputum.
4. Sweating, cyanosis, and tachycardia.
5. Moist sounds on chest auscultation.
6. Pulsus paradoxus.

Investigations

1. **Chest X-ray**:
    a. Pulmonary congestion, and interstitial edema. Karley B lines.
    b. White out appearance of lung fields.
2. **Hemodynamic studies**:
    a. Increased CVP. Elevated jugular venous pressure
    b. Increased pulmonary capillary wedge pressure
    c. Increased right atrial pressure
    d. Decreased cardiac output.
3. **Electrocardiogram**:
    a. Signs of ischemia, infarction, and arrhythmias
    b. Left atrial or ventricular enlargement.
4. **Arterial blood gas studies**:
    a. Decreased PaO_2 increased $PaCO_2$
    b. Decreased pH.
5. Total blood count.
6. Blood biochemistry and electrolytes.
7. Urine analysis.

Management

1. Promote adequate oxygenation. Maintain a clear patent airway. Tracheobronchial toilet. IPPV may be necessary.
2. Cardiac workload should be reduced by alleviating anxiety and tension.
3. Strict bed rest. Elevate patient's head and chest. It will decrease venous return to heart and lungs.
4. Judicious administration of morphine is always helpful. Respiratory depression should be avoided.
5. Frusemide IV—It is a diuretic, venodilator and it decreases pulmonary congestion.
6. Venodilators like nitroglycerin may also be needed as it augments the effect of frusemide.

7. Aminophylline is helpful as it relieves bronchospasm and has weak diuretic and inotropic effects.
8. Pulmonary capillary pressure may be reduced by mechanical means. Soft rubber tourniquets may be applied in one extremity, allowing arterial perfusion, but restricting venous flow. This should be rotated every 15 minutes to the free extremity. Phlebotomy and removal of 250–500 ml blood may be done in some selected cases.
9. Continuous monitoring of vital signs, ECG, hemodynamic studies, arterial blood gas study, chest X-ray, etc. are essential.
10. Antiarrhythmic drugs: Lignocaine, quinidine, and procainamide.
11. Inotropic agents: Digoxin, dobutamine, dopamine. These drugs increase cardiac output, increase cardiac contractility, reduce preload, and pulmonary capillary wedge pressure. Optimize myocardial contractility.
12. Parenteral arterial dilators may be indicated in cases of hypertension and valvular insufficiency. Nitroprusside is particularly useful.
13. Precipitating factors such as arrhythmias, hypertension, etc. should be judged and managed accordingly.
14. Surgical intervention may be indicated in cases of valvular insufficiency.
15. Myocardial depressant drugs should be avoided. Avoid hypervolemia, hypovolemia, hypotension, hypokalemia, and hypoxemia.
16. Nutritional care to prevent negative nitrogen balance.

Complications

1. Hypoxemia.
2. Hypokalemia.
3. Hypovolemia and shock due to profound diuresis or reduction of preload.

Hypertensive Crisis

A hypertensive crisis may be arbitrarily defined as an abrupt increase of diastolic pressure above 130 mmHg with clinical manifestations of specific organ damage. It may be associated with congestive cardiac failure, encephalopathy and/or oliguria. This is a life-threatening condition and the hypertensive state must be reduced within hours to prevent severe organ damage or even death.

Usually, these patients have essential hypertension along with secondary illness. There is chronic vasoconstriction of the arterioles along with atherosclerotic condition of vessels resulting an increased peripheral or systemic resistance. Extremely high blood pressure may lead to acute myocardial infarction, cerebrovascular accident, liver failure, renal failure, and any other vital organ failure.

Precipitating/Associated Conditions

1. Chronic essential hypertension.
2. **Renal hypertension**: Acute glomerular hypertension, renovascular hypertension. Renal tumors.
3. Eclampsia.
4. Pheochromocytoma, Cushing's disease.
5. **Cardiovascular disorders**: Acute myocardial infraction, acute left ventricular failure, pulmonary edema. Fluid overload.
6. **Neurologic disorders**: Head injury, spinal cord injury, cerebrovascular accident, subarachnoid hemorrhage.
7. **Drug interaction**: Cocaine, LSD, tricyclic antidepressants. Withdrawals of antihypertensive drugs.
8. Administration vasopressor medications.

Clinical Findings

1. Headache, anxiety, visual impairment, nausea/vomiting, numbness, tingling, and palpitations.
2. *Neck vein distension*: Altered consciousness, peripheral edema, papilledema and raised blood pressure.

Investigations

1. Complete blood count.
2. Blood biochemistry: Urea and creatinine increased.
3. Plasma catecholamine level increased in pheochromocytoma.
4. Urine vanillylmandelic acid increased in pheochromocytoma.
5. Chest X-ray.
6. Electrocardiogram.
7. CT scan and MRI in selected cases.
8. Urine output.

Management

1. Maintain bed rest. Ensure adequate oxygenation and ventilation.
2. Relieve anxiety and tension.
3. Monitor vital signs and ECG.
4. Cardiac monitoring.
5. Continuous blood pressure monitoring.
6. Check peripheral pulse frequently.
7. Drug therapy:
    a. Sodium nitroprusside, nitroglycerine and diazoxide.
    b. Trimethaphan camsylate IV.
    c. α-adrenergic blocking agents: Phentolamine.
    d. β-adrenergic blocking agents: Propranolol, esmolol, and labetolol.
    e. Calcium channel blockers: Nicardipine and verapamil.

f. Angiotensin-converting enzyme inhibitors.
g. Diuretics: Frusemide.

Complications

1. Myocardial ischemia/infarction—Arrhythmias.
2. Congestive cardiac failure—Pulmonary edema.
3. Hypertensive encephalopathy—Cerebral hemorrhage.
4. Raised intraocular tension.

Shock

Shock may be defined as a state of generalized inadequacy of tissue perfusion to meet the oxygen demand of the tissues resulting impaired cellular metabolism and if not therapeutically intervened progressing to multiple organ failure and even death. Hypotension itself is a fall in arterial blood pressure of more than 20% below normal or an absolute value of systolic pressure below 90 mmHg or of MAP below 60 mmHg.

Classification

1. **Hypovolemic shock**: Loss of circulating fluid volume. Loss of blood volume. Hemorrhage and fluid loss.
2. **Cardiogenic shock**: Poor pumping ability of heart. Myocardial infarction, acute arrhythmia, heart failure, severe heart valve lesion, pericardial tamponade, pulmonary embolism, and tension pneumothorax.
3. **Neurogenic shock**: Generalized vasodilation and loss of vasomotor tone causing massive increase in vascular capacity and decreased venous return to heart. Spinal cord injury and reflex vasodilation.
4. **Anaphylactic shock**: An antigen antibody reaction resulting release of histamine and histamine-like substance with dilation of venous and arterial system and loss of fluid into tissue spaces.

5. **Septic shock**: Generalized infection of blood mostly by gram-negative bacteria resulting marked vasodilation, peripheral pooling of blood and decreased systemic vascular resistance as in cases of bacteremia, septicemia.

Causes

1. **Decreased blood volume**: Hemorrhage, massive injury, severe vomiting, severe diarrhea, cholera, and burns dehydration.
2. **Poor pumping action of the heart**: Acute myocardial infarction, acute arrhythmias, pericardial tamponade, cardiomyopathy, pulmonary embolism, tension pneumothorax, etc.
3. **Neurogenic causes**: Spinal cord injury.
4. **Anaphylactic shock**: Hypersensitivity to foreign proteins, pollen, insect stings, etc. Adverse drugs reactions and mismatched blood transfusion.
5. **Septic shock**: Bacteremia, septicemia, and endotoxemia.

Stages of Hemorrhagic Shock

1. **Initial stage, stage of compensation**: Initially, there are transient decrease in blood volume, reduction of cardiac output and fall of arterial blood pressure. These stimulate the responses of sympathetic nervous system to increase their activities. Renin-angiotensin aldosterone responses are activated to compensate and prevent further fall of blood pressure. Vasomotor center increases its activity and thereby increases peripheral resistance and raises blood pressure. Increased secretion of adrenaline, noradrenaline, glucocorticoids, mineralocorticoids, antidiuretic hormone (ADH) and renin also occur. There may be

reduced output of urine and reduced skin, muscle, renal, splanchnic, and coronary blood flow.
2. **Stage of shock, intermediate stage**: When compensatory mechanisms fail to maintain the effective blood pressure, the patient will be in state of shock. There are progressive fall of blood pressure, decreased blood flow to the vital organs like brain, heart, diaphragm, skeletal muscles, and so on. Venous return and central venous pressure fall and hence cardiac output and tissue perfusion suffer. Excessive tachycardia and profound hypotension occur. These may lead to myocardial ischemia and heart failure. Profound renal vasoconstriction along with excessive secretion of ADH may ultimately lead to oliguria and anuria. Profound metabolic acidosis occurs in shock. Coagulopathy, pulmonary edema and adult respiratory distress syndrome may also be seen in late stage of shock.
3. **Stage of irreversible shock**: In this stage the patient becomes unresponsive to active efficient treatment and condition gradually deteriorates. Constricted resistance vessels become unresponsive to catecholamines. It is mostly due to profound hemodynamic instability and cellular hypoxia leading to underperfusion and ischemic anoxia to vital organs. Myocardial depression, failure of vasomotor center, extensive tissue damage and multiple organ failure are evident in late stage of shock.

Clinical Features

Clinical features mostly depend on the etiology, type, and severity of the shock. History of traumatic injury, infection, cardiac illness, etc. may be there.
1. *Extremities*: Cool.

2. *Sensorium changes*: Apathy, agitation, and coma.
3. *Pupils*: Dilated and reactive or with sluggish reaction.
4. Tachycardia and pulse feeble: Arrhythmias. Diminished heart sounds.
5. *Blood pressure*: Low, cannot be recorded in severe cases.
6. Tachypnea.
7. Thirst and nausea/vomiting.
8. Urine output low.
9. Body temperature low.
10. Muscle weakness.
11. Skin cold and clammy, but may be warm and flushed in septic shock.
12. Signs of hypoxia, and cyanosis may be present.

Cardiogenic Shock

It is a severe form of pump failure and it may indicate 35%–40% loss of functioning myocardium. Profound hypotension occurs, systolic pressure is often less than 80 mmHg and mean blood pressure is less than 60 mmHg. Extreme oliguria (urine less than 500 ml/24 hours) may occur. There is elevated filling pressure. Pulmonary edema occurs due to left ventricular failure.

Investigations

1. **Arterial blood pressure**: Low and a systolic pressure of less than 60 mmHg is often associated with vital organ hypoperfusion.
2. **Central venous pressure**: Low CVP of less than 5 cm. H_2O indicates hypovolemia.
3. **Hematocrit and hemoglobin estimation**: Low hematocrit value may indicate blood loss. It may increase in cases of hemoconcentration.

4. **Total blood count**: WBC count increased in septic shock.
5. Serum lactate increases.
6. **Arterial blood gas analysis**: Decreased pH in metabolic acidosis.
7. **Urine analysis**: Urine volume low. Specific gravity increases.
8. Blood culture and sensitivity test are helpful in cases of septic shock.
9. Electrocardiogram.
10. Serum electrolytes and creatinine.
11. **Pulmonary artery pressure**: Pulmonary capillary wedge pressure.
12. Chest X-ray.
13. Pulse oximetry.

Management

- Early diagnosis and immediate care are essential for successful management.

Primary aims

A. *To treat hypovolemia*: Fluid and volume replacement. Blood, plasma, and plasma substitutes.
B. *To improve impaired tissue perfusion*: Steroids and inotropic drugs.
C. *To combat infection*: Antibiotics.
D. *To improve metabolic changes*:
   1. Fluid and volume replacement:
      a. Early restoration of intravascular fluid volume.
      b. Plasma expanders—Crystalloids and colloids.
      c. Blood transfusion—Blood and blood products.
   2. The patient should be kept supine with legs slightly elevated 15°–20°. Hemorrhage should be arrested. Basic lesion should be treated.

3. Adequate oxygenation and ventilation: Patent airway should be maintained. Adequate ventilation. Supplemental oxygen. IPPV with 100% oxygen in extreme cases.
4. Monitoring the vital signs is essential. Blood pressure, CVP, hemodynamic parameters, urinary output, determination of skin/core temperature, blood gas analysis, serial hemoglobin, packed cell volume, and electrolyte estimation need careful monitoring.
5. Sodium bicarbonate to treat metabolic acidosis. THAM may also be used.
6. Vasodilators may be used to improve the amount of available oxygen for tissues. Phenoxybenzamine, phentolamine and chlorpromazine can be used. But these should be used with adequate precautions and proper monitoring.
7. Inotropic drugs: Dopamine and dobutamine improve myocardial contractility, increase cardiac output and arterial blood pressure, and organ perfusion.
8. Sympathomimetic drugs like noradrenaline, adrenaline, methoxamine, phenylephrine, etc. may raise blood pressure by causing vasoconstriction. Vasopressors may have to be repeated as necessary to maintain an acceptable blood pressure.
9. Steroid therapy is controversial in treatment of shock. Steroids have α-adrenergic blocking action, stabilizing action on arterial walls and may protect the patient from endotoxic and anaphylactic shock. Steroid therapy is only indicated when conventional vasoactive drugs have failed to improve the state of shock. Steroid therapy should be continued for 72 hours and no tailing off is needed.

10. Digitalis may be indicated when associated with tachycardia, atrial fibrillation or flutter in elderly patients.
11. Antibiotics are indicated in septic shock preferably after culture and sensitivity test.
12. Surgical treatment may be necessary to treat injury, localized collection of pus as in cases of bacteremic and hemorrhagic shock.
13. Vagolytic drugs like atropine sulfate are needed particularly in neurogenic shock associated with bradycardia.
14. Shock associated with myocardial infarction needs special attention.
    a. Primary pump failure—Treatmet of cardiogenic shock:
        i. Relief of pain—Analgesics.
        ii. Oxygenation.
        iii. Correction of acidosis.
        iv. Correction of dysrhythmias.
        v. Volume replacement should be judicious.
        vi. Inotropic agents—Isoprenaline, salbutamol, and dopamine.
        vii. Mechanical balloon counterpulsation.
    b. Dysrhythmias: Drug therapy, cardioversion, and pacemaker.
    c. Mechanical complications may need surgery as in acquired septal defect, ventricular aneurysms, etc.
    d. Other cardiopulmonary causes like cardiac tamponade, pulmonary embolism, pneumothorax and dissecting aneurysms need special treatment accordingly.
15. General supportive care:
    a. Establish central IV line.

b. Maintain fluid and electrolyte balance, acid-base balance.
c. Adequate oxygenation and tissue perfusion.
d. Monitor vital signs, hemodynamic status, ECG, acid-base changes, electrolyte changes, fluid volume replacement and for coagulopathy.
e. Nutritional care and metabolic support.
f. Prevent and control of infections.
16. Prevent other life-threatening complications. These should be treated accordingly, whenever needed:
a. Disseminated intravascular coagulation
b. Adult respiratory distress syndrome
c. Acute renal failure
d. Cardiorespiratory failure
e. Hypothermia
g. Multisystem organ failure
h. Congestive heart failure and pulmonary edema from excessive fluid administration
i. Cerebral ischemia and cerebral edema.

Note

Signs of adequate intravascular fluid replacement:
1. Heart rate is less than 100 beats/min.
2. Pulse pressure is more than 30 mmHg.
3. Urinary output is within 0.5–1 ml/kg/hr.
4. No metabolic acidosis.
5. Effects of positive pressure ventilation on blood pressure is little.

Cardiac Tamponade

Cardiac tamponade or pericardial tamponade is the accumulation of fluid or blood in the closed pericardial cavity limiting ventricular filling, causing low cardiac output and resulting in hemodynamic compromise. It is a life-threatening emergency and needs urgent care and treatment.

Causes

1. Bleeding after cardiothoracic surgery. Clot obstruction of mediastinal chest drain.
2. Perforation/penetrating injury of the heart.
3. Injury of a coronary artery or myocardium during cardiac catheterization or cardiac biopsy.
4. Following myocardial infarction and myocardial wall rupture.
5. Coagulopathy, patients with anticoagulants or fibrinolytic therapy.
6. Pericardial infection.
7. Pericardial malignancy.
8. Following radiation therapy to the mediastinum.
9. Chronic renal failure and uremia.
10. Rheumatologic/autoimmune diseases.
11. Ruptured aortic aneurysm with bleeding in the pericardial cavity.

Diagnosis

1. **Chest X-ray**: Increased size of the cardiac silhouette. Note that cardiac silhouette on a chest radiography may not change until about 250 ml of fluid is present in the pericardial space.
2. **Echocardiography**: Fluid accumulation in pericardial cavity.
3. **Hemodynamic monitoring**:
    - Central venous pressure—Increased
    - Pulmonary artery pressure—Increased
    - Pulmonary capillary wedge pressure—Increased
    - Cardiac output—Low.

4. **Electrocardiogram**: Low voltage ECG—Arrhythmias
5. **Pericardial fluid examination**: Culture and sensitivity test.

Note

1. The pericardial cavity usually contains 20–30 ml of fluid. The sac is fixed and fibroserous in nature and minimally distensible. The sac surrounds the heart and great vessels.
2. The pericardium has a low compliance and the speed of air, fluid or blood accumulation dictates the degree of decline in cardiac performance and rapidity of onset of symptoms.
3. A rapid increase of an additional 150–200 ml of fluid can critically compromise myocardial function. If it accumulates slowly, symptoms may not occur even if volume is 1 liter or more.

Clinical Manifestations

1. Midthoracic chest pain, dyspnea and shortness of breath, apprehension, and restlessness.
2. Increased central venous pressure.
3. Activation of sympathetic system: Tachycardia and vasoconstriction.
4. Decreased cardiac output.
5. Narrow pulse pressure—Pulsus paradoxus (systemic blood pressure decreases less than 10 mmHg during inspiration).
6. Profound systemic hypotension.
7. Muffled heart sounds and weak tachycardiac pulse.
8. Neck vein distension.
9. ECG: Electrical alternans (alternating large and small QRS complexes or altered direction of complexes). Decreased voltage.

10. Atrial filling pressures and pulmonary end-diastolic pressure are mostly equal at a relatively high value, about 20 mmHg.

Differential Diagnosis

1. Pulmonary embolism.
2. Tension pneumothorax.
3. Right ventricular failure.
4. Right ventricular myocardial infarction.
5. Constrictive pericarditis.
6. Acute aortic dissection.

Management

Prevention

1. Adequate surgical care and hemostasis during cardiothoracic surgery.
2. Careful placement of intracardiac monitoring devices and pacemaker leads.
3. Treat medical problems, if any.
4. Treat coagulopathy, if present.

Treatment

1. Early diagnosis and prompt management are necessary.
2. Careful monitoring is essential particularly following cardiothoracic surgery and placement of CVP line and pulmonary artery catheter.
3. *Drug therapy*:
   a. Adequate oxygenation.
   b. Measures to maintain stroke volume:
      i. Expansion of intravascular fluid volume.
      ii. Inotropic agents: Isoprenaline, dobutamine, dopamine, and adrenaline.

iii. Sodium bicarbonate for correction of metabolic acidosis.
iv. Atropine sulfate may be needed to reverse bradycardia due to vagal reflexes.
v. Diuretics may also be needed.
c. Percutaneous subxiphoid pericardiocentesis. A negative tap is possible in presence of large blood clots compressing the heart.
d. Pericardiotomy.
e. Emergency thoracotomy and rapid evacuation of blood may sometimes be lifesaving.

Complications

1. Cardiac arrest—Electromechanical dissociation.
2. Acute heart failure.
3. Myocardial ischemia/infarction.
4. Infection.
5. Trauma/injury of heart and/or lungs during pericardiocentesis.

Management of Anesthesia

1. Intrapericardial pressure should be relieved before induction of anesthesia, whenever possible.
2. If it is not possible to relieve intrapericardial pressure, adequate care must be taken to maintain cardiac output.
3. Avoid bradycardia. Maintain heart rate in between 90 and 140 beats per minute.
4. Avoid anesthesia-induced decreases in myocardial contractility and systemic vascular resistance.
5. Hypovolemia should be corrected and filling pressure should be optimized to compensate for anesthesia-induced vasodilation.

6. Induction of anesthesia may be done with IV ketamine.
7. Succinylcholine is helpful for rapid intubation.
8. Use of ketamine, midazolam, and fentanyl is mostly satisfactory. Avoid volatile anesthetics and some IV anesthetics known to cause myocardial depression.
9. Avoid vigorous positive pressure ventilation of lungs as it may further reduce venous return.
10. Continuous monitoring of CVP, systemic blood pressure, and ECG is essential.
11. Emergency pericardiocentesis may have to be done, if circulatory collapse occurs at the time of induction.

Chapter 3

Neurologic and Central Nervous System Disorders

Head Injury

Head injury may be defined as craniocerebral trauma due to injury of skull or brain or both. It is mostly due to a motor vehicle accident, a fall or a direct impact on head and is frequently associated with other injuries such as cervical spinal injury, thoracoabdominal injury and so on.

Head injury may have certain types and basic pathophysiology are as follows:

1. **Closed head injury**: No penetration of the skull and skull cavity not exposed to external environment.
2. **Open head injury**: Cranial contents exposed to external environment.
3. **Coup injury**: Injury of brain directly at the site of impact.
4. **Contrecoup injury**: Injury of brain opposite to the site of impact.
5. **Diffuse injury**: Injury involved the entire brain.
6. **Primary impact damage**: It is mostly due to accleration/deceleration forces applied to the skull contents. There may be contusions of the cortex both beneath the site of impact and contrecoup affecting widely in the brain.

7. **Secondary head injury**: It is due to hemorrhage and edema. Intracerebral and subdural bleeding may occur at the time of injury. Hematoma within the rigid skull may result to increased intracranial pressure and brain shift. Infection may also occur.

    Increased intracranial presure can also cause decreased cerebral perfusion pressure and ischemia of the brain.

8. **Skull fractures**:
    a. Linear fracture: Crack in the skull.
    b. Comminuted fracture: Fragmentation of skull bones.
    c. Depressed fracture: An inward depresion of skull fragments. Compound fracture may be associated with infection.
    d. Basilar skull fracture: Fracture of the base of the skull. It may be associated with bleeding into the nasopharynx with the consequent danger of inhalation of clots. It carries a high risk for cerebrospinal leakage and infection through a dural tear in the ear or nose.

9. **Extradural hematoma**:
    a. History of a blow to the temporal region with loss of consciousness. It is followed by a lucid interval and then again unconsciousness.
    b. Increasing drowsiness, dilatation of pupil on the affected side and hemiparesis on opposite side.
    c. Apnea, other pupil dilates and death occurs.
    d. Evacuation of blood clot through a burr hole is the lifesaving treatment.

10. **Cerebral edema**: Following trauma, there may be cerebral edema increasing gradually. It is usually associated with increased intracranial tension, increasing coma, fixed dilated pupils, and ultimately respiratory failure.

11. **Changes in cerebral hemodynamics**: Localized brain injury produces local tissue acidosis and vasodilation. These blood vessels become unresponsive to changes in arterial PCO_2 as in normal areas of brain. The effect of hypercarbia is thus to cause vasodilation in normal areas of brain and divert blood from the damaged areas which have a luxury perfusion. Loss of local autoregulation resulting in 'steal phenomenon' if there is hypoxia, hypercarbia, and hypotension. Treatment with IPPV results in hypocapnia and the reverse situation develops. Intracranial pressure is reduced and blood is diverted to perfuse the damaged brain tissue.
12. Brainstem injury interferes with the vital centers and may cause decerebrate rigidity and hyperthermia.
13. **Airway obstruction**: It may be due to unconsciousness, and falling back of tongue, associated injuries such as fracture of mandible or fracture of roof of pharynx resulting in hemorrhage in the pharynx and depression of reflexes and thus more risk of aspiration. Airway obstruction causes straining, hypoxia, and hypercarbia and thus raised intracranial tension.
14. Cardiovascular collapse.
15. Damaged brain cannot tolerate minor insults, fat embolism, hypoxia, hypercarbia, and hypotension.
16. Acute head injury is frequently associated with other injuries including cervical spine and thoracoabdominal injuries. These need careful attention.

Clinical Assessment

1. A full history of trauma.
2. General physical examination. Any other significant trauma.
3. Neurological examination: Mental status, skull and spine need careful examination.

4. Headache, tingling, paresthesia, and paralysis.
5. Level of consciousness: Fully conscious, confusion, lethargy, stupor, and coma. Rising ICP may often be associated with papilledema and rapidly deteriorating conscious level.
6. Any dysfunction of cranial nerves.
7. The Glasgow coma scale is a standardized scale, accepted all over to assess the severity of head injuries. It is based on eye opening, verbal, and motor response (Table 3.1). Each response on the scale is given a number, high for normal and low for impaired response.

Table 3.1: The Glasgow coma scale

Sign	Evaluation	Score
Eye opening	Nil	1
	To pain	2
	To speech	3
	Spontaneous	4
Verbal response	Nil	1
	Garbled	2
	Inappropriate	3
	Confused	4
	Oriented	5
Motor response	Nil	1
	Extension	2
	Abnormal flexion	3
	Flexion withdrawal	4
	Localizes pain	5
	Obeys	6

The lowest score is 3 and maximum is 15. The responsiveness of the patient is indicated by the total number obtained. In severe head injury a score may be 7 or less.

8. Size and reaction of pupil:
   a. Pinpoint: Pontine hemorrhage and narcotic overdose.
   b. Small: Drug-related, metabolic coma, and pontine hemorrhage.
   c. Midposition and nonreactive: Midbrain damage.
   d. Dilated bilateral and fixed: Severe anoxia, and death.
   e. Pupil shape—Ovoid or slightly oral: Increased ICP; irregular in trauma to the pupil.
9. Convulsion.
10. Leakage of CSF: Basilar skull fracture.
11. Other findings: Bradycardia and abnormal respiration. Rising blood pressure and falling pulse rate indicate rising ICP.
12. Hyperthermia.
13. Abnormalities in motor function: Paresis, paralysis, abnormal gait, and involuntary movements.

Investigations

1. Skull X-ray.
2. Computed tomography: It is helpful to detect epidural hematoma, subdural hematoma, intracranial shift, herniation, etc.
3. Magnetic resonance imaging: Posterior fossa lesions and brainstem lesions.

Management

1. **Establishment and maintenance of airway and adequate ventilation**:
   a. Cleaning of airway, tracheobronchial toilet, and care of oropharyngeal airway.
   b. Endotracheal intubation and IPPV.
   c. Tracheostomy may be needed.
   d. Fracture of cervical spine may be associated. Laryngoscopy and intubation or any head movement

may be dangerous in such cases. An axial or in-line manual traction should be applied throughout.
2. **Resuscitation of cardiovascular collapse**: IV infusion of fluids, colloids or blood may be indicated. Vasopressors, and dopamine may be helpful for fluid and electrolyte balance.
3. **Assessment and management of associated injuries**: Facial trauma, neck trauma, and chest injury may be there.
4. **Monitor and promote neurologic functions**: Monitoring of vital signs is essential.
5. **Supportive treatment**:
   a. Indwelling urinary catheter.
   b. Nasogastric tube.
   c. IV infusion of fluids.
   d. Nutrition: Parenteral nutrition may be indicated.
   e. CVP or pulmonary artery catheter is essential for hemodynamic monitoring.
   f. Skin care.
   g. Prevention and treatment of infection: Antibiotics.
   h. Chest physiotherapy.
6. Reduce or prevent increased ICP:
   a. Dexamethasone.
   b. Osmotic diuretics.
   c. Hyperventilation.
7. **Control and prevention of convulsions**:
   a. Anticonvulsants: Diazepam, phenytoin, and phenobarbitone.
8. **Management of complications**:
   a. Hyperthermia.
   b. Coma.
9. Consultation with other specialists like neurosurgeon, etc. may be indicated.

Cerebrovascular Accident

Cerebrovascular accident refers to an area of brain damage resulting from a circulatory disturbance such as thrombosis, embolism or hemorrhage. It may be either minor with recovery to normal or major with severe and permanent disability or even death.

Causes

1. **Cerebral thrombosis**:
   a. Essential hypertension with atherosclerosis.
   b. Hypotension as following myocardial infarction.
   c. Inflammatory diseases of blood vessels such as temporal arterities, polyarteritis nodosa, systemic lupus erythematous, etc.
   d. Hematological disorders: Polycythemia.
   e. Use of oral contraceptives.
2. **Cerebral embolism**:
   a. Mitral valve disease with atrial fibrillation.
   b. Prosthetic heart valve.
   c. Subacute bacterial endocarditis.
   d. Fat, air or malignant cells.
3. **Intracranial hemorrhage**: It may be either cerebral or subarachnoid.
   a. Rupture of small arterioles or microaneurysms.
   b. Rupture of a congenital aneurysm.
   c. Mycotic aneurysm caused by weakening of the arterial wall around a septic emboli.
   d. Arteriovenous aneurysms.
   e. Anticoagulant therapy.

Diagnosis

1. Computed tomography
2. Lumbar puncture

3. Cerebral angiography
4. Hematologic studies
5. Blood biochemistry
6. Chest radiography
7. ECG.

Management

1. General management and nursing care of an unconscious patient.
2. **Supportive measures**:
    a. Bed rest and sedation.
    b. Respiratory care, tracheobronchial toilet, adequate oxygenation, and IPPV.
    c. IV infusion, fluid electrolyte balance, and nutrition.
3. Monitoring of vital functions is essential.
4. **Steroids**: Dexamethasone.
5. Hypertension should be controlled.
6. **Specific treatment**:
    a. Cerebral thrombosis or embolism:
        i. Anticoagulant therapy.
        ii. Aspirin.
    b. Cerebral embolism:
        i. Control of atrial fibrillation.
        ii. Treatment of subacute bacterial endocarditis.
    c. Cerebral hemorrhage:
        i. Reduction of raised intracranial tension.
        ii. Aminocaproic acid.
        iii. Calcium channel blockers to reduce cerebral vasospasm.
        iv. Surgical management.

Cerebral Edema

Cerebral edema implies the swelling of the brain mass mostly either due to accumulation of water or brain congestion. There is an increase in brain water content both in intracellular and extracellular compartments. Intracellular fluid accumulation generally occurs in gray matter and extracellular fluid accumulation is mainly in white matter.

Types

1. **Vasogenic**: It is due to disruption of blood-brain barrier as in cases of trauma, ischemia, pressure effect of space occupying lesion, malignant arterial hypertension, etc. Extent and spread of vasogenic edema is mostly determined by the site of lesion, size of vascular leak and pressure force to move the fluid outwards.
2. **Hydrostatic**: Here the cerebral edema is mostly due to high cerebrovascular transmural pressure.
3. **Cytotoxic**: The usual causes are ischemic hypoxia, local ischemia due to intracranial vascular lesion, general systemic ischemia affecting the whole brain, bactericidal agents like hexachlorphene, etc. Here the edema is mostly widespread with severe intracranial tension.
4. **Interstitial**: It is usually of obstructive in nature as in high pressure hydrocephalus.
5. **Hypo-osmotic**: If plasma osmolality is reduced by 12%, there may be brain edema with rise of intracranial pressure. Here the cell membrane is intact and water alone shifts from the vascular compartment following an osmotic gradient.

Clinical Features

1. History of head injury
2. Hypoxia

3. Coma: Level of consciousness gradually declines
4. Focal signs of hemispheric disturbance must develop
5. Fixed dilated pupil and respiratory failure.

Investigations

1. CT scan.
2. Cerebral angiography.
3. Lumbar puncture.
4. Assess ICP through an extradural pressure transducer and calculate cerebral perfusion pressure (CPP).
   CPP = Mean arterial pressure – ICP.
5. Blood biochemistry, serum electrolytes, blood gas analysis, chest radiograph, ECG, etc. are often helpful.

Management

1. Primary aim should be to reduce the intracranial hypertension, to restore brain distortion and shift, and to increase cerebral blood flow in regions of ischemia.
2. General supportive measures:
   a. Adequate oxygenation—IPPV.
   b. IV fluids and vasopressors.
   c. Care of the unconscious patient.
   d. Care of the skin, eyes, bowel, and bladder.
   e. Normal body temperature should be maintained.
   f. Antibiotics to treat infection.
   g. Nutritional care.
   h. Monitor the vital signs, and ICP.
3. Hypoxemia should be treated promptly. Adequate oxygenation and ventilatory assistance are needed. Tracheostomy is often helpful.
4. Arterial perfusion should be maintained with systolic pressure between 110 and 140 mmHg. Hypotension causes further ischemia and hypertension augments brain edema.

5. Specific measures:
   - Dehydration therapy.
     a. Hyperventilation: Moderate hypocapnia is always beneficial to reduce cerebral blood flow and thereby lower the ICP.
     b. Hypertonic solutions:
        i. IV 20% mannitol.
        ii. 50% glucose.
        iii. Urea.
     c. Steroids: It reduces brain water content, reduces ICP and brain shift, and improves cerebral blood flow.
     d. Diuretics: Frusemide.
6. Monitoring of vital signs and blood biochemistry, estimation of serum electrolytes, ECG, blood gas analysis, and frequent neurological assessment are essential to determine the prognosis and for better therapeutic management.

Status Epilepticus

Status epilepticus is a clinical condition characterized by rapid repetitive recurrence of any type of seizure without recovery between attacks. It constitutes a grave risk of life by causing airway obstruction, hypoxia, and consequent cerebral damage and cardiac arrhythmia. Seizures may occur alone or as a clinical manifestation of other diseases. However, generalized tonic-clonic or grand mal seizures which are convulsive, are the most dangerous.

Causes

1. Noncompliance or inadequate dosage of anticonvulsants in cases of known epilepsy.
2. Sudden withdrawal of anticonvulsant drugs.

3. Brain tumor (often frontal lobe) and cerebral abscess.
4. Head injury/cerebrovascular disease/encephalitis/meningitis.
5. Liver/kidney disease.
6. Metabolic disorders:
   a. Hypoglycemia
   b. Hypercarbia
   c. Decreased cerebral oxygen
   d. Electrolyte imbalance
   e. Acid-base imbalance.
7. Withdrawal or overdose of some drugs: Phencyclidine, and cocaine.
8. Alcohol withdrawal.

Pathophysiology

Seizures are produced by abnormally hyperactive neurones which form an epileptogenic focus, rapidly and repeatedly depolarizing the cells involved. These may remain localized or spread throughout the entire cortex. Oxygen and nutritive sources are exhausted. The body tries to compensate with an increase in cerebral blood flow. With repeated seizures, low blood glucose level and oxygen content occur. Anaerobic metabolism starts and cellular lactate levels increase. All these complicate the condition of the patient.

Clinical Findings

1. **Aura phase**: The patient feels uneasiness, visual or auditory sensation which may occur several hours or even days before the actual seizure. Nausea and confusion may occur.
2. **Tonic phase**: Consciousness decreases with excessive muscular contraction and even apnea can occur. Pupils become dilated and nonreactive to light.

3. **Clonic phase**: Patients become more violent with jerking movements, often accompanied by forceful, rapid and deep respirations, eyes roll back, profuse sweating and salivation.
4. **Recovery phase**: Muscles become flaccid, consciousness returns, exhaustion, headache and fatigue, confused and lethargic, pupillary reaction becomes normal.

Investigations

1. Total blood count
2. Urine analysis
3. Serum electrolytes
4. Blood glucose estimation
5. Blood biochemistry, urea, and NPN
6. Serum SGOT and SGPT
7. Arterial blood gas analysis
8. Serum lactate level
9. Electroencephalogram
10. Computed tomography scan
11. Lumbar puncture and CSF analysis
12. Monitoring of ICP.

Management

Primary aim should be to secure airway, protect the patient from injury, drug therapy to control convulsion and to maintain fluid and electrolyte balance.

1. **Precautionary measures for seizure patients**:
   a. Bed rest and place bed in low position.
   b. Suction equipment should be available.
   c. Oxygen equipment and emergency resuscitation equipment should be kept ready.
   d. Monitor vital signs frequently.

e. IV line should be there. Treat dehydration and electrolyte imbalance.
   f. Cardiac monitor is often helpful.
   g. Adequate oxygenation, IPPV, and tracheobronchial toilet. Respiratory resuscitation.
   h. EEG monitoring may be necessary.
   i. Monitor body temperature. Cooling may be necessary, if temperature increases.
   j. Avoid drugs which may activate epileptic foci. Methohexitone, enflurane, and ketamine should not be used.
2. **Drug therapy**:
   a. Diazepam IM or IV 10–20 mg
   b. Paraldehyde IV 0.1 mg/kg
   c. Phenytoin 100–200 mg IV
   d. Clonazepam
   e. Chlormethiazole, carbamazepine, and valproic acid
   f. Sedatives: Pentobarbital
   g. Lignocaine upto 5 mg/kg IV
3. Monitor and assess possible injury. Provide for patient safety. Assess neurological signs after seizure.
4. General anesthesia and curarization, endotracheal intubation, and artificial ventilation may be attempted in severe cases. The therapy is meant for patients who do not respond to conventional treatment. Muscle relaxants alone do not interfere with continuous firing of neurons.

Poliomyelitis

Poliomyelitis is an acute infective disease due to an enterovirus which have a predilection for the anterior horn cells of spinal cord and the motor nuclei of the brainstem. The virus can be cultured from the stools and nasopharynx of the patient during the active and convalescent stages.

Clinical Features

1. Initial phase of viremia: Slight fever, general malaise, sore throat, minor gastrointestinal upset, and flu-like illness.
2. Second phase starts a few days after infection. Virus invades the central nervous system. Symptoms are those of a viral meningitis. Pain, paresthesia, tenderness of muscles, weakness and then paralysis.
3. Paralytic phase occurs within 24–72 hours of the second phase of illness. A lower motor neuron lesion occurs. Any muscle or a group of muscles may be affected. Involvement of the bulbar muscles is dangerous as it may result aspiration and respiratory insufficiency. Paralysis progresses for upto 72 hours.
4. Recovery is often delayed and may sometimes be incomplete.

Diagnosis

1. Viral studies in CSF and stool.
2. CSF examination: In early stages, excess polymorphs, moderate rise of protein; but in late stage, lymphocytes predominate.
3. Arterial blood gas analysis: Hypoxia and hypercarbia.

Management

1. No specific treatment for poliomyelitis.
2. Prevention is possible by oral polio vaccine.
   - 1st dose
   - 2nd dose: 8 weeks after 1st dose
   - 3rd dose: 8–12 months after 2nd dose
   - Additional dose: On entering school.
3. Monitor respiratory function and assess airway patency.

4. IPPV: Adequate oxygenation.
5. Supportive measures: Total bed rest and nutritional care. Fluid and electrolyte balance.
6. Physiotherapy only after recovery. Paralysis may become worse, if affected muscles are exercised during the phase of progression of the paralysis.
7. Promote physical and motor strength in arms, legs, feet, and hands.

Tetanus

Tetanus is a disease of central nervous system caused by the toxin produced by *Clostridium tetani*. The organism is anaerobic and the spores are widely found in soil, dust, and general environment. The organism multiplies only under anaerobic conditions. Its neurotoxin, tetanospasmin is produced as the organism multiplies and attacks the central nervous system after an incubation period of 7–10 days. The incubation period may vary and range from 2–52 days.

- The neurotoxin inhibits the release of acetylcholine at the neuromuscular junction while suppressing inhibiting internuncial neurons in the central nervous system. The disease is characterized by generalized (occasionally localized) muscle spasm by the neurotoxin.

Clinical Features

1. Pain and spasm of jaw muscles.
2. Trismus.
3. Pain and stiffness in the back and neck. Pain is often aggravated by movement.
4. Facial spasm of risus sardonicus.
5. Dysphagia.

6. Laryngospasm.
7. Convulsion.
8. Respiratory embarassment.
9. Cardiovascular instability, hyperpyrexia, paralytic ileus, and gastric dilatation.
10. Bulbar palsies and facial palsy.
11. Increased sympathetic system activity, tachycardia, and hypertension.
12. In severe cases, spasm becomes more frequent and may even be continuous. Every muscle goes into spasm and respiration ceases.
13. Depending upon the severity of infection, the clinical picture may vary. With successful treatment, the spasms improve gradually and full recovery is possible.

Prophylaxis

1. Everyone should be properly immunized with tetanus toxid.
2. In cases of injury some measures are to be taken:
   a. Wound debridement and aseptic dressing.
   b. Antibiotic cover: Long-acting penicilin, tetracycline, erythromycin, etc.
   c. Tetanus toxoid.
   d. Antitetanus toxin.

Treatment

Primary aim should be directed to remove the source of toxin, to neutralize toxin not yet fixed to nervous system, to maintain adequate ventilation and to control muscle spasm.

1. Complete bed rest in dark and quiet room. Adequate medical and nursing supervision is essential.
2. Wound debridement and aseptic dressing.
3. Use of systemic antibiotics.

4. Toxin neutralization with human antitetanus immunoglobulin.
5. Adequate sedation: Chlorpromazine, promethazine, diazepam, chlordiazepoxide, and chloral hydrate.
6. Diazepam relieves muscle spasm. In severe cases, neuromuscular blocking agents may be needed with IPPV.
7. Maintenance of respiratory function. Adequate oxygenation, mechanical ventilation, and IPPV.
    a. Patent clear airway
    b. Tracheostomy may be needed
    c. Tracheobronchial care and toilet may be needed
    d. IPPV.
8. Convulsions should be controlled by barbiturates, paraldehyde, bromethol, or diazepam.
9. Nutritional care: Parenteral feeding and tubefeeding.
10. Maintain fluid and electrolyte balance.
11. Maintain acid-base balance.
12. Infection should be treated with antibiotics.
13. Hyperpyrexia may occur and it should be tackled carefully.
14. Cardiac dysrhythmia: Lignocaine and adrenergic blockers may prove useful.
15. Hypotension: IV infusion of fluids and vasopressors.
16. Careful monitoring of vital signs is essential. ECG monitoring is often helpful.
17. Painful tonic contractures may require analgesic drugs.
18. Mortality rate is high and thus measures for prophylaxis are most important. Complete recovery may take several months. Physiotherapy may be needed during that phase of recovery.

Increased Intracranial Pressure

Increased intracranial pressure (ICP) implies sustained pressure greater than 15 mmHg within the cranial cavity. It is also termed as intracranial hypertension. A sustained intracranial pressure greater than 20 mmHg is known as malignant intracranial hypertension.

Causes

1. Head injury.
2. Cerebral hematoma and tumors.
3. Subarachnoid hemorrhage, cerebral edema due to infection, hypoxia, trauma, etc.
4. Hydrocephalus.
5. Craniostenosis.
6. Arterial dilation from any cause.
7. Venous obstruction from any cause.

Pathophysiology

Cranial cavity contains brain tissue, blood, and CSF. It has a fixed volume and there is only one exit through foramen magnum. An increase in its contents may change ICP. However, some compensation may occur by decreasing CSF and blood volume. But when those mechanisms have been overcome, ICP rises above the normal range 5–13 mmHg.

Brain tissue volume increases due to tumors or cerebral edema. Cerebral edema is due to an increase in the water content in brain tissue.

Cerebral blood volume (CBV) is mostly controlled by the venous system. Under a limited regulatory mechanism when a hematoma or tumor causes an increase in ICP, the CBV is displaced to compensate; but upto a certain limit and after that limit, a small increase in lesion size may cause a great increase in ICP.

Cerebral blood flow is mostly dependent on cerebral autoregulation, cerebral perfusion pressure, cerebral metabolic rate of $PaCO_2$ and PaO_2. Cerebral blood flow is directly related to the cerebral perfusion pressure (CPP) and cerebrovascular resistance. CPP represents the difference between mean arterial pressure and intracranial pressure. Normal CBF is 45–65 ml/100 gm of brain tissue per minute. CPP should not be allowed below 50–60 mmHg to support brain function.

CBF is maintained at a constant level by a compensating autoregulation which operates within a mean arterial pressure 60–150 mmHg. Above 150 mmHg, the blood-brain barrier is disrupted resulting in cerebral edema. Autoregulation affects the brain by maintaining arterial pressures by vasoconstricting or vasodilating arterioles in response to systemic pressure. It also affects in response to rise in $PaCO_2$ and to low $PaCO_2$.

Cerebrospinal fluid volume may increase due to overproduction, abnormality in circulation drainage, and reabsorption.

Increased systemic blood pressure produces increased CBF and intracranial blood volume leading to increased ICP when autoregulation fails.

Decreased systemic blood pressure causes decreased CBF and intracranial blood volume resulting in low oxygen content in brain, brain ischemia with subsequent brain edema.

- **Blood gases**: Acidosis or low oxygen level in blood causes vasodilation of cerebral arteries and subsequent ischemia and edema of brain. Respiratory alkalosis or low $PaCO_2$ caused by hyperventilation leads to vasoconstriction of cerebral arteries and subsequent ischemic brain damage.

- Hyperpyrexia increases cerebral metabolic demand. If metabolic needs are not adequately provided, ischemia will occur. It is said that 1°C rise of temperature causes 7%–10% increase in cerebral metabolic demand.

Clinical Features

1. Headache, nausea, and vomiting.
2. Increased blood pressure and bradycardia.
3. Transient impairment of vision and diplopia.
4. Alteration in the level of consciousness.
5. Papilledema and fixed dilated pupils.
6. Seizure activity.
7. Herniation of brain tissue is due to pressure gradient. Location of the area of high pressure determines the nature of herniation.
   a. Diencephalic herniation: It is caused by a medial supratentorial lesion that forces the diencephalon through the tentorial notch. Clinical findings include Cheyne-Stokes respiration, small but reactive pupils and paresis of upward gaze and altered mental status.
   b. Uncal herniation: It is caused by a lateral supratentorial lesion that forces the uncus (medial portion of temporal lobe) through the tentorial notch. It produces alteration of consciousness, a dilated unreactive pupil ipsilateral to the mass from 3rd cranial nerve compression and hemiparesis on either side.
   c. Tonsillar herniation: It is due to pressure that forces the inferior portion of cerebellum through the foramen magnum compressing the medulla. Alteration of consciousness, irregular breathing, and even apnea may occur.

- Medullary coning may cause damage to spinal tracts by mechanical pressure. The obstruction of foramina of Magendie and Luschka will lead to further rise of ICP. This causes a vicious cycle and becomes irreversible. Convulsion can occur.
8. Hydrocephalic cry in infants.
9. If CSF pathways are not obstructed, the raised ICP is reflected in a high CSF pressure in lumbar puncture.

Diagnostic Tests

1. ICP monitoring
2. Computed tomography scan
3. Magnetic resonance imaging
4. Brain scan
5. EEG
6. Cerebral angiogram
7. ECG
8. Serum electrolytes estimation
9. Total blood count
10. Urine analysis.

Problems of Raised ICP

1. Very susceptible to depressant drugs, narcotic drugs, anesthetics, etc.
2. Chances of failure of vital functions due to critically lowered perfusion to vital centers.
3. Brain is edematous.
4. Medullary coning and fatal results may occur.

Management

1. Adequate oxygenation. Ventilatory assistance and IPPV.
2. Arterial blood gas studies should be done frequently. Pulse oximeter is always helpful. Oxygen saturation should be monitored.

3. Cerebral venous drainage should be promoted. Head of the bed should be elevated 20°–30°.
4. Maintain normothermia.
5. Care of the eyes, bowel, and bladder.
6. Tracheobronchial toilet with gentle adequate care. Preoxygenation is often helpful.
7. Maintain fluid and electrolyte stability.
8. Nutritional care.
9. Prevention of aspiration of gastric contents: gastric tube is often needed.
10. Neurosurgical treatment is the definitive treatment for some causes of raised ICP such as epidural, subdural, and cerebellar hematoma.
11. Neurosurgical intervention is not recommended for increased ICP following ischemic, anoxic or metabolic brain necrosis. Some measures and drug therapy are employed to decrease ICP.
    a. Posture: Avoid head down position.
    b. Hyperventilation: $PaCO_2$ should be maintained 25–30 mmHg.
    c. Drainage of CSF: Drain through ventriculostomy or lumbar subarachnoid catheter.
    d. Hyperosmotic drugs: Mannitol 0.25–1 gm/kg IV.
    e. Diuretics: Frusemide 1 mg/kg IV.
    f. Corticosteroids: It may relieve localized cerebral edema as in cases of trauma, abscess, and hemorrhage. Edema due to anoxia or infarction does not respond to steroids.
12. In cases of brain herniation, forced hyperventilation and osmotic diuretics are useful, but these are temporary measures able to delay advancing herniation.
13. Treat the complications, if any.

a. Herniation syndrome: It is a downward protrusion of the brain from the cranial cavity through the tentorium due to increased intracranial pressure.
   i. Monitor the change of behavior: Restlessness.
   ii. Deterioration of level of consciousness: Coma.
   iii. Note any change of respiratory pattern: Cheyne-Stokes respiration, irregular breathing, and apnea.
   iv. Note pupillary size and reaction: Sluggish to nonreactive dilated pupils. Bilaterally fixed dilated pupils in late stage.
   v. Assessment of motor response: Hemiparesis, hemiplegia, ipsilateral rigidity, decerebrate posturing, flaccidity with occasional decerebrate movements in late stage.
b. Serial seizures: Anticonvulsants, phenytoin, and phenobarbitone.
c. Malignant intracranial hypertension: It is characterized by a sustained ICP more than 20 mmHg resulting ischemia and neuronal damage. Monitor vital signs and neurologic studies continuously. Emergency resuscitation is mandatory.
d. Hyperpyrexia: Maintain body temperature near normal, cooling, and antipyretics.
e. Hypertension: Antihypertensive drugs and sodium nitroprusside may often be helpful.

Brain Death

Brain death may be defined as an irreversible condition occurring when the entire brain and brainstem cease to function. When brain death is confirmed, then only it is possible to terminate artificial ventilation and other mechanical supports provided the existing law permits.

Diagnosis of Brain Death

1. **Presence of coma**: The cause of coma, apnea and brain damage is known as irreversible.
2. Reversible causes such as hypothermia, drug intoxication, metabolic and endocrine disturbances must be excluded. There should be no profound disturbance of serum electrolytes, acid-base balance and/or blood sugar concentrations.
3. **Apnea**: Spontaneous respiration must have ceased and the patient is on artificial ventilation. Muscle relaxants and other drugs must be excluded as a cause of respiratory failure. No respiratory movements must occur even when $PaCO_2$ is allowed to rise 7 kPa as measured by a arterial sampling. In practice, the patient is ventilated with 100% oxygen for 10 minutes followed by 5% carbon dioxide in oxygen for 5 minutes. Ventilator is then disconnected for 10 minutes while oxygen is insufflated to trachea at 6 L/min. There will be no spontaneous respiration in case of brainstem death.
4. **Brainstem reflexes must be absent**:
    a. Pupils are fixed usually at midpoint. Nonreacting to light stimuli.
    b. No corneal reflex.
    c. No motor responses to skin stimulation anywhere within the cranial nerve stimulation.
    d. Absent gag reflex: No pharyngeal reflex or responses to the stimulus of tracheal suction.
    e. Absent vestibulo-ocular reflex: 20 ml of ice-cold water is instilled onto the eardrum. No movement of the eye in response indicates brainstem death.
    f. Oculocephalic reflex: Turn the patient's head from side to side and observe eye movements. Eyes do not move (China doll) in nonfunctioning brainstem.

Eyes move (swivel-eyed doll) in functioning brainstem.
5. **Spinal reflexes**: Spinal reflexes can be present even when brain death has occurred.
6. **Electroencephalography**: Isoelectric EEG.
7. **Cerebral angiography**: Absent cerebral circulation.
   - The assessment should be repeated after at least 4 hours for confirmation of brainstem death. The observation should be done in presence of at least two consultants preferably neurosurgeon, neurophysician, anesthe-siologist, and ITU physician in charge.

Guillain-Barré Syndrome

It is defined as an acute or subacute motor and sensory polyneuropathy. The etiology is unknown; but it may be due to secondary to an allergic phenomenon affecting the peripheral nerves. The onset may be after an unspecified viral or bacterial infection or febrile illness or vaccination. Infective mononucleosis, measles, psittacosis or mycoplasmal infections are mostly associated with the disease.

The disease is thought to be a demyelination of the cranial and spinal peripheral nerves caused by an autoimmune reaction that causes destruction of myelin sheath encircling the nerves. It results in obstruction of both motor and sensory impulses and the syndrome produces muscle weakness and paralysis. The cranial nerves (facial nerve, glossopharyngeal nerve, vagus, spinal accessory, and hypoglossal nerve) may also be affected.

1. Ascending type is most commonly seen with motor and sensory deficits progressing from distal extremities to the cranial nerves. It affects both sides equally and the patient becomes quadriplegic.

2. Descending type affects the cranial nerves first and then in the periphery. Respiratory involvement is common in early stage.
3. Pure motor Guillain-Barré syndrome is mostly like ascending type, but no sensory involvement is noted.

Clinical Features

1. There may be hypersensitivity, numbness, and tingling sensation in hands and feet.
2. Headache, stiff neck, photophobia, and muscle cramps.
3. Bilateral muscle weakness progressing to paralysis.
4. Weakness often starts distally and advances centrally with respiratory involvement.
5. Inability to smile, frown, close eyelids, speak, and swallow or chew.
6. Hypotension and cardiac arrhythmia.
7. Paralytic ileus.
8. Urinary retention.

Investigations

1. **Analysis of CSF**: Increased protein levels; cell count mostly normal.
2. Arterial blood gas study.
3. **Electromyography**: Decreased nerve conduction.

Management

1. Monitor respiratory function and arterial blood gas study. Assess hypoxia/hypercarbia.
2. **Adequate oxygenation**: Tracheobronchial toilet, endo-tracheal intubation and IPPV.
   Tracheostomy may be needed.
3. **Supportive treatment**: Monitor vital signs and cardiac monitor is often helpful.

4. **IV line**: Pulmonary catheter.
5. Fluid and electrolyte balance.
6. **Nutritional care**: Promote nutritional/fluid status.
7. Maintain urinary catheter drainage.
8. Drug therapy is controversial. Steroids may be given.
9. **Prevention of infection**: Antibiotics.
10. Vasopressors may be indicated in cases of hypotension.
11. Prevention of aspiration.
12. Promote mobility and strength of muscles.
13. Physiotherapy to the limbs is essential to prevent wasting and contractures.

Coma

Coma is characterized as a sleep-like state of unresponsiveness to external stimulation. This state of brain failure may be due to various metabolic and structural disorders.

Causes

1. **Intracranial disorders**: Head injury, meningitis, encephalitis, cerebrovascular accident, subarachnoid hemorrhage, epilepsy, cerebral malaria, cerebral edema, etc.
2. **Metabolic disorders**: Hypoglycemia, uremia, diabetes, respiratory failure, hepatic failure, myxedema, hypothermia, and anoxia.
3. **Poisoning**: Overdose of narcotics, barbiturates, alcohols, exposure to toxins, venoms, etc.

Pathophysiology

1. Usually coma results from the lesion affecting both cerebral hemispheres or the brainstem. Lesions affecting only one single hemisphere usually does not cause coma, but with their mass effect can cause

coma as in cases with tumor, hemorrhage, or massive infarction by causing compression to opposite side of brain and brainstem.
2. Cerebellar lesions can cause unconsciousness by causing compression on brainstem.
3. Brainstem lesions cause coma by causing disruption of reticular formation.
4. Metabolic diseases impair consciousness by effects on the reticular formation and/or both cerebral hemispheres.

Differential Diagnosis of Coma

It depends on meticulous assessment of history, general physical examination, neurologic examination, and some investigations.

1. **History**: History is the most important. History of trauma, use of drugs, toxin exposure, pre-existing illness such as liver disease, kidney disease, diabetes, epilepsy, etc. may establish a diagnosis. Friends, relatives, and even neighbours can help in this matter.
2. **General physical examination**: It may reveal the pre-existing medical illness.
3. **Neurological examination**: A thorough neurologic examination should be made. Repeated examinations at intervals are needed to evaluate the course of the disease.
   a. Level of consciousness: Reaction to painful stimuli.
   b. Pupil size and reaction to light: Midposition and fixed pupils may denote midbrain lesion. Unilateral dilated and fixed pupil may imply oculomotor nerve lesion. Small but reactive pupils usually seen in narcotic overdose, metabolic encephalopathy or pontine lesions. Bilateral dilated and fixed pupil occurs in severe anoxic encephalopathy or in overdose with glutethimide or scopolamine.

c. Papilledema may suggest a rise in ICP, in some drug overdose and carbon dioxide narcosis.
d. Dysconjugate gaze occurs in cranial nerve palsy. Oculomotor nerve palsy causes deviation of the eye laterally and inferiorly, but a sixth nerve lesion causes deviation of the eye medially.
e. Conjugate deviation of the eyes towards the hemiparetic side results from a pontine lesion opposite the side to which the eyes look, and away from the hemiparetic side suggests the lesion above the pons on the side to which eyes look.
f. Absence of all eye movements may suggest bilateral pontine lesion and some drug overdoses as with sedatives, phenytoin, and tricyclic antidepressants.
g. Oculocephalic maneuver: It is tested by quickly turning the head laterally and watching the eyes. Normally, the eyes move conjugately in the opposite direction and it suggests that the brainstem pathways with the pons and midbrain are intact.
h. Caloric stimulation: Ice-cold saline 10–30 ml is poured on the tympanic membrane, the eyes conjugately deviate without nystagmus toward the ear being stimulated, when the brainstem from pons to medulla is intact.
i. Motor responses: Spontaneous movements should be assessed for symmetry and purposiveness. Response to painful stimulation should be observed. Muscle tone, deep tendon reflexes, and pathologic reflexes like Babinski's sign need careful observation. Neck stiffness may be present.
4. Any associated injury, scalp injury should be examined.

Investigations

1. Total blood count: Hb% and WBC.

2. Blood biochemistry: Urea, NPN, sugar, and creatinine.
3. Serum electrolytes.
4. Liver function tests.
5. In cases of poisoning full toxicological examinations.
6. Blood gas studies.
7. Skull X-ray, and cervical spine radiograph.
8. Lumbar puncture and examination of CSF.
9. Echoencephalography to detect any midline shift.
10. EEG.
11. Isotope imaging.
12. Neuroradiology: Angiography may be indicated in cases of subdural hematoma, space-occupying lesions, and cerebral aneurysms.
13. Computed tomography.

Management

1. Certain measures should need immediate attention even while assessing the patient:
   a. Monitor and promote respiratory integrity. Adequate maintenance of clear patent airway. Tracheobronchial toilet. Adequate oxygenation. Mechanical ventilation—IPPV. Observe precautions to avoid aspiration.
   b. Monitor and promote cardiovascular function. IV infusion of fluids, fluid and electrolyte balance. Vasopressors.
   c. Maintain normal body temperature.
   d. Increased intracranial pressure should be treated. Hyperventilation, mannitol infusion, and frusemide.
   e. Dextrose infusion to treat hypoglycemia.
   f. Naloxone is the antidote of opioid overdose.
   g. Underlying cause should be identified and managed accordingly. Surgical intervention may be needed.

h. Patients should be treated in ICU, where all sorts of facilities and monitoring equipment, etc. are available.
2. General care of unconscious immobile patients:
   a. Nutritional care.
   b. Fluid and electrolyte balance, and acid-base balance.
   c. Proper positioning. Prevention of cutaneous pressure sores.
   d. Joint mobility should be maintained.
   e. Care of the eyes, and prevention of corneal abrasions.
   f. Maintain urinary drainage catheter patency to prevent urinary tract infections or bladder distension.
   g. Antacids may be needed for prevention of gastrointestinal hemorrhage.
   h. Heparin may be indicated to prevent deep vein thrombosis.

Traumatic Spinal Cord Injury

Spinal cord injury can result from various causes such as motor vehicle accidents, sports injuries, violence, falls, trauma, etc. Most spinal cord injuries involve the cervical spine, usually between C_4–C_7, Spinal cord injuries can cause complete quadriplegia. These patients may have associated with traumatic head injury and injuries to other organs.

Clinical features:

1. Spinal shock with flaccid are flexic paralysis and lack of all sensations.
2. Airway problems and ventilatory insufficiency.
3. Hypotension and circulatory insufficiency. Hypovolemic and neurogenic shock can co-exist.
4. Instability of the spine.

Neurologic and Central Nervous System Disorders

Immediate care

This is most important even before neurologic evaluation.
1. Establishment of adequate airway.
2. Adequate ventilation of lungs.
3. Endotracheal intubation should be done by using manual in line immobilization. Flexion of neck must be avoided. Fiber optic intubation may be helpful.
4. Circulatory support: Fluid administration, vasopressors.
5. Associated injuries also need adequate care.
6. Patient should be placed in a scoop stretcher or similar back board with supportive blocks. Straps should be used to prevent uncontrolled movements. Patients with suspected cervical spine injury rigid collar immobilization is mandatory. Improper positioning of unstable spine can cause increased intracranial tension, airway compromise, diminished chest wall mobility, pressure, sores, and pain. Patient should be transported very cautiously to a definitive trauma treatment center.

Neurologic Evaluation

1. Standard neurologic examination including assessment of mental status, cranial nerves, motor sensory testing, and reflex testing.
2. Multiple view radiography.
3. Computed tomography.
4. Magnetic resonance imaging (MRI).
5. Myelography.

Spinal Column Injuries

These are bone or ligamentous disruptions of the spinal column. These can occur in bone fractures or ligamentous instability. In such cases compression and injury of neural elements can result. However, spinal column injury can occur without spinal cord injury and vice versa. It should be noted that spinal cord injury and spinal column injury are distinct separate entities and these can exist together.

Causes of Spinal Cord Disorder

1. Trauma: Compression fractures
2. Degenerative: Disk herniation
3. Infection: Myelitis, abscess, tuberculosis, etc.
4. Inflammatory and demyelinations: Transverse myelitis, multiple sclerosis, etc.
5. Tumors/metastases
6. Vit B_{12} deficiency
7. Syringomyelia
8. Spondylosis
9. Stenosis of spinal canal.

Various syndromes are being described where pathologic criteria correlate to anatomical areas of injury. These help to localize the level of injury.

1. **Posterior cord injury**: Loss of proprioception/vibration sense (posterior columns), preservation of motor and pain, and temperature. It is usually nontraumatic. It may be due to vitamin deficiency and infections such as syphilis.
2. **Central cord injury**: It can occur in patients who are in excessive motion in sagittal plane (hyperextension/hyperflexion) particularly those with pre-existing cervical stenosis. Here the central part of the spinal cord suffers necrosis due to vascular compromise. There is impairment of hands and arms more than legs, bladder dysfunction and variable degrees of sensory loss below the level of the injury.

3. **Anterior cord injury**: It is mostly due to spinal artery occlusion with resultant loss of all motor and sensory function except proprioception and vibration.
4. **Hemisection spinal cord (Brown-Séquard syndrome)**: There is loss of ipsilateral motor and proprioception/vibration with contralateral loss of pain and temperature, two to three segments below the level of injury.
5. **Complete transaction**: There is complete loss of bilateral motor and sensory function below the level of injury.
6. **Conus medullaries syndrome**: It is usually less painful, symmetric, upper motor neuron affection with varying degree of weakness, sensory loss, bladder, bowel, and sexual dysfunction.
7. **Cauda equina syndrome**: It results from a compressive lesion below the level of spinal cord. It causes saddle paresthesia, weakness of legs, bowel and bladder dysfunction. Early surgical decompression is advised for maximal recovery and prevention of further damage.

Management

1. Patient should be treated in definitive trauma/critical care center.
2. Prevention of secondary cord injury is mandatory. Hypotension, shock, hypoxia hypercoagulability and hyperthermia can cause further deterioration.
3. Adequate oxygenation and ventilation.
4. Treat shock and hypotension, fluid replacement, and vasopressors may be needed.
5. Detailed radiographic studies, computed tomography, and MRI are helpful to confirm the diagnosis.
6. Pain relief: Analgesics.

7. High doses of steroids.
8. Prevention of deep vein thrombosis and pulmonary embolism: Unfractionated or low-molecular-weight heparin is helpful.
9. General supportive care, prevention of gastroparesis, ileus, stress ulcers, and gastrointestinal bleeding: H_2 antagonists and proton pump inhibitors. Prevention of pressure ulcers.
10. Neurosurgery consultation.
11. Surgical intervention.
12. Postoperative rehabilitation.

Nontraumatic spinal cord disorder (myelopathy):
1. Most patients do not require admission in critical care unit.
2. Some patients particularly with involvement of upper cord may have the risk of respiratory insufficiency and cardiovascular instability. They need supportive care and resuscitative measures as usual.
3. Some cases need surgical intervention such as resection of abscess, high dose of steroids or IV immunoglobulin for inflammatory diseases.

Myasthenia Gravis

It is an autoimmune disease of the motor-end plate. It causes a functional decrease in acetylcholine receptors of the neuromuscular junction. Symptoms and signs are characterized by periods of exacerbation and remission.

Clinical Features

1. Ptosis and diplopia are most common symptoms in initial stage.
2. Weakness of most commonly used muscles; pharyngeal and laryngeal muscles, dysphagia, facial

weakness with chewing and speaking, asymmetric skeletal muscle weakness.
3. May be associated with thymus tumors, cardiomyopathy, rheumatoid arthritis, systemic lupus erythematosus, and thyroid disorders.
4. Short-acting anticholinesterase drugs can transiently increase the strength of the muscles.
5. Electromyography and nerve conduction studies and elevation acetylcholine receptor antibody assay are helpful to confirm the disease.

Management

1. Anticholinesterase drugs: Pyridostigmine
2. Corticosteroids
3. Immunosuppressant drugs
4. Plasmapheresis
5. Thymectomy in selected cases
6. Avoid aminoglycosides and other medications those lead to exacerbation.

Medications that can aggravate muscle weakness in myasthenia gravis:
A. Certain antibiotics: Aminoglycosides, ciprofloxacin, erythromycin, azithromycin tetracyclines, etc.
B. Antiarrhythmic drugs: Quindine, lignocaine, procainamide, β-blockers, and calcium channel blockers.
C. Neuromuscular blocking agents: Vecuronium, pancuranium, and suxamethonium,
D. Miscellaneous: Lithium, phenytoin, and quinine.

Cholinergic Crisis

It can occur from an excess of acetylcholine at nicotinic and muscarinic sites. It is usually due to excess anticholinesterase administration.

Clinical Features

Muscle weakness, wheezing, increased salivation and secretions, muscle fasciculations, nausea, vomiting, diarrhea, lacrymation, bradycardia, dysphagia, aspiration pneumonitis, hypotension, respiratory insufficiency, and respiratory failure.

Cholinergic crisis should be carefully differentiated from myasthenic crisis. Pupil is dilated in myasthenic crisis but constricted in cholinergic crisis. Edrophonium improves muscle power in myasthenic crisis but no change in muscle power or exacerbation of symptoms in cholinergic crisis.

Management

1. Adequate oxygenation and ventilation.
2. Endotracheal intubation and controlled ventilation in cases with respiratory failure.
3. Muscarinic side effects of cholinergic crisis should be treated with atropine or glycopyrrolate.

Chapter 4

Liver Diseases

Acute Liver Failure

Acute liver failure may be defined as a clinical syndrome associated with massive necrosis of liver cells or with sudden severe impairment of liver functions. This may occur in a previously normal liver or in cases with chronic liver disease such as cirrhosis of liver.

Causes

1. **Previously normal liver**:
    a. Viral hepatitis.
    b. Drugs like paracetamol, halothane, and carbon tetrachloride.
2. **Pre-existing liver disease**: Cirrhosis of liver, hepatic vein thrombosis, and chronic hepatitis.
    Precipitating factors:
    a. Gastrointestinal hemorrhage.
    b. Infection.
    c. Over diuresis.
    d. Surgery, anesthesia.
    e. Paracentesis.
    f. Alcohol.

g. Misuse of drugs like acetaminophen overdose, antidepressants, anticonvulsants, sulfonamides, amiodarone, trimethoprim and sulfamethoxazole combination, etc.
h. Ischemia: Cardiac failure, shock, and hypoxemia.
i. Metabolic disorders: Acute fatty liver. Wilson's disease, pregnancy, etc.

Pathophysiological Considerations

1. **Hepatic encephalopathy**:
   a. Inability to detoxicate nitrogenous substances derived from gastrointestinal protein breakdown by the damaged liver.
   b. Cerebral edema.
   c. Acid-base disorders.
   d. Depletion of neurochemical transmitters.
   e. Increased levels of short-chain fatty acids.
2. **Coagulopathy**:
   a. Decreased clotting factors.
   b. Abnormal platelet production and function.
   c. Intravascular coagulation (tissue thromboplastin from necrotic liver cells).
   d. Abnormal vessel fragility.
3. **Jaundice**:
   a. Decreased survival of red blood cells.
   b. Inability of the liver to metabolize bilirubin.
4. **Increased susceptibility to infection**:
   a. Impaired immunity.
   b. Impaired function of liver cells on leukocytes.
5. **Cardiovascular changes**:
   a. Vasodilation and hypovolemia.
   b. Increased cardiac output.
   c. Stimulation of sympathetic nervous system.

6. **Pulmonary changes**:
   a. Intrapulmonary shunting.
   b. Mismatched ventilation perfusion ratio.
   c. Hypoxemia.
7. Hepatorenal failure.
8. **Cerebral edema**: Vasogenic or cytotoxic.
9. Hypoglycemia.
10. Metabolic acidosis.
11. **Electrolyte changes**: Hypokalemia and hyponatremia.

Clinical Manifestations

1. Headache, dizziness, agitation, violent delirium, mania, somnolence, and sudden coma.
2. Jaundice and nausea/vomiting.
3. Fetor hepaticus, tachypnea, and respiratory insufficiency.
4. Hypotension, tachycardia, arrhythmia, and cardiac failure.
5. Body temperature increased.
6. Grading of hepatic encephalopathy:
   a. Grade 1: Mood change and confusion
   b. Grade 2: Drowsy and abnormal behavior
   c. Grade 3: Stupor and rousable
   d. Grade 4: Unrousable even by painful stimulation.
7. Bleeding manifestations, purpura, bruising, and bleeding from gastrointestinal tract.
8. Features of pre-existing liver disease: Clubbing, spider naevi, palmar erythema, splenomegaly, and ascites.
9. Metabolic disorders:
   a. Hypoglycemia.
   b. Electrolyte changes: Hypokalemia.
   c. Acid-base changes:
      i. Hypokalemia—Metabolic alkalosis.
      ii. Hyperventilation—Respiratory alkalosis.
      iii. Tissue necrosis—Metabolic acidosis.
      iv. Lactic acidosis is most common.

Laboratory Investigations

1. Blood sugar: Hypoglycemia
2. Serum electrolytes: Hypokalemia and hyponatremia
3. Blood urea nitrogen: Decreased
4. Coagulation studies: Thrombocytopenia, increased prothrombin time and partial thromboplastin time
5. Screening for hepatitis
6. Serum bilirubin: Increased
7. Liver function tests: Increased serum SGOT, SGPT, and alkaline phosphatase
8. Complete blood count
9. Serum ammonia: Increased
10. Arterial blood gas analysis: Hypoxia and acidosis
11. Urine analysis (granular cast, blood); urine electrolytes,
    a. Urine sodium—Decreased
    b. Urine osmolality—Increased
12. EEG
13. ECG
14. Chest X-ray: Pulmonary edema and aspiration pneumonitis
15. CT scan of liver
16. Ultrasonography of liver.

Management

1. **General measures**: Precipitating factors, if any, should be detected and corrected as far as practicable. Hypoxia, hypotension, and hypovolemia should be treated. Bleeding from esophageal varices should be managed. CVP monitoring is essential. Blood transfusion may be needed. Blood should be as fresh as possible. No sedatives or hypnotics or hepatotoxic drugs should be given. Complete bed rest. Foolproof nursing care. Adequate oxygenation. Insertion of a

nasogastric tube may be beneficial. Monitoring of vital signs and laboratory findings are essential.

2. **Appropriate measures for hepatic encephalopathy**:
   a. Diet: Restriction of protein intake. About 1500–2000 calories/day should be needed. Glucose may be given through gastric tube or intravenously.
   b. Antibiotics may be given to reduce intestinal bacterial flora and thus to reduce absorption of nitrogenous substances. Neomycin is the preferred drug.
   c. Enema or purgation.
   d. Oral lactulose—Osmotic laxative.
   e. No sedative/hypnotic/narcotic drugs. It is dangerous to prescribe these drugs in patients with acute liver failure.

3. **Control of metabolic disturbances**:
   a. Hypoglycemia: IV infusion of glucose solution. Monitoring of blood glucose level at 12–hour interval.
   b. Hypokalemia and alkalosis is best treated with potassium chloride replacement. Frequent electrolyte estimation is needed. Any imbalance should be corrected.
   c. Hyponatremia is often corrected with fluid restriction. IV saline is avoided.
   d. Acid-base balance should be maintained.
   e. Renal failure: It may be either acute tubular necrosis or renal failure with low urine sodium concentration. Uremia causes coma, aggravates bleeding tendency and increases the risk of infection. Frusemide may be helpful. Peritoneal dialysis is the preferred treatment.

4. **Hemorrhagic manifestations**:
   a. Avoid arterial punctures. Avoid nasal intubation.
   b. Parenteral vitamin K.
   c. Fresh frozen plasma and platelet packs.

    d. Fresh blood transfusion.
    e. Gastrointestinal bleeding should be controlled. Cimetidine should be given even if there is no clinical signs of bleeding.
 5. Maintain blood pressure and cardiac output.
 6. Volume overload should be avoided. Pulmonary edema needs early detection and management.
 7. **Temporary liver support**:
    a. Exchange blood transfusion.
    b. Hemoperfusion using activated charcoal may be tried.
    c. Liver transplant.

Common Complications

 1. Renal failure
 2. Infection
 3. Hemorrhage
 4. Pancreatitis
 5. Pulmonary edema
 6. Respiratory failure.

Chronic Hepatic Failure

Chronic hepatic failure is usually characterized by the slow, gradual, and progressive degeneration of liver cells resulting in diminished liver function and ultimately liver failure.

Causes

 1. Cirrhosis of liver is most common in:
    a. Alcoholic
    b. Postnecrotic cirrhosis
    c. Biliary cirrhosis
    d. Cardiac cirrhosis.
 2. Chronic hepatitis

3. Budd-Chiari syndrome
4. Nodular regenerative hyperplasia.

Pathophysiological Considerations

1. Portal hypertension.
2. Vascular spiders: Palmar erythema.
3. Testicular atrophy, gynecomastia, and menstrual irregularity.
4. Anorexia and poor health.
5. Hypoalbuminemia.
6. Jaundice.
7. Coagulopathy.
8. Fetor hepaticus.
9. Hypovolemia, vasodilation, and hypotension.
10. Pulmonary changes: Intrapulmonary shunting, mismatched ventilation perfusion ratio, and hypoxemia.
11. Increased tissue protein breakdown.
12. Increased susceptibility to infection.
13. Hepatic encephalopathy: Disordered consciousness, altered neuromuscular activity. Precipitating factors include azotemia, misuse of opioid sedative hypnotic drugs, gastroesophageal hemorrhage, constipation, high protein diet, etc (Table 4.1).

Table 4.1: Grading of encephalopathy

Grade	Metal state	EEG
Grade 1	Confusion, euphoria altered mood/behavior	Normal
Grade 2	Drowsy	Generalized slowing
Grade 3	Stuporous but rousable	Delta activity
Grade 4	Comatose, responds to pain	Triphasic waves
Grade 5	Deep comatose	Flat

Clinical Manifestations

1. Malaise, weakness, loss of body weight, fatigue, anorexia, and nausea/vomiting.
2. Vascular spiders, palmar erythema, edema, ascites, spleen enlarged, tachycardia, hypotension, tachypnea, little rise of body temperature, gynecomastia, menstrual irregularities, and fetor hepaticus. Liver may be enlarged or decreased.
3. *Complications*:
   a. Gastrointestinal bleeding
   b. Infection
   c. Hepatorenal syndrome
   d. Gross electrolyte imbalance.
4. Severity of the liver disease can be assessed by modified child's grouping (Table 4.2).

Table 4.2: Modified child's grouping			
Prognostic scoring	**Score 1**	**Score 2**	**Score 3**
Encephalopathy	None	Gr. I and 2	Gr. 3, 4, 5
Bilirubin mmol/L	< 25	25–40	> 40
Albumin g/L	35	28–35	< 28
Prothrombin time secs prolonged	1–4	4–6	> 6
Ascites	Absent	Slight	Moderate

Score less than 6 denotes good risk. 7, 8, 9 denotes moderate risk. More than 10 is poor risk.

Investigations

1. Blood sugar level—Decreased.
2. Serum electrolytes—Decreased sodium, potassium, and phosphate.
3. Blood urea nitrogen—Decreased.

4. Coagulation studies—Platelet count decreased, prothrombin time increased.
5. Hepatitis screening test.
6. Serum bilirubin—Increased.
7. Liver function test—SGOT, SGPT, alkaline phosphatase increased.
8. Serum albumin—Decreased.
9. Complete blood count.
10. Serum ammonia—Increased.
11. Serum lactic acid—Increased.
12. Arterial blood gas analysis—Hypoxemia.
13. Urine analysis—Urine sodium decreased, increased protein, granular cast, blood present, increased specific gravity and osmolality.
14. EEG.
15. ECG.
16. Chest X-ray.
17. CT scan of liver.
18. Ultrasonography of liver.
    - Common extrahepatic problems in fulminant liver disease—
    a. Cerebral: Hepatic encephalopathy and cerebral edema.
    b. Pulmonary: Intrapulmonary shunting and hypoxemia.
    c. Cardiac: Hyperdynamic state and cardiomyopathy.
    d. Renal: Increased ACTH and aldosterone activity, water retention, and impaired ability to concentrate urine.
    e. Electrolyte and acid-base changes.
    f. Hemostasis: Thrombocytopenia and DIC.

Management

1. **Hepatic encephalopathy**:
   a. Restriction of protein intake. Vegetable protein may be used. Branched-chain amino acids are better tolerated.

b. All sedative, hypnotics, opioids, and narcotics should be avoided.
　　c. Removal of fecal matter from colon—Laxatives and enemas.
　　d. Lactulose orally, lactulose enema, and phosphate enema.
　　e. Neomycin may be given orally or through nasogastric tube.
　　f. Prevent dehydration and avoid using nephrotoxic drugs and diuretics aggressively.
　　g. Treat hypokalemia.
　　h. Prevention and treatment of gastrointestinal bleeding, systemic infection, diarrhea, and constipation.
　　i. IV glucose for nutrition.
　　j. Charcoal hemoperfusion, hemodialysis, and liver transplant.
2. **Coagulopathy**:
　　a. Monitoring of coagulation studies.
　　b. Fresh frozen plasma, platelets, and vitamin K.
3. **Ascites and edema**: It is mostly due to sodium retention by the kidney, decreased plasma osmotic pressure, increased splanchnic lymph flow and raised hydrostatic pressure in liver sinusoids and portal vein.
　　a. Salt restriction and water restriction.
　　b. Bed rest.
　　c. Diuretics—Spironolactose, frusemide, and thiazides.
　　d. Paracentesis.
　　e. Salt-free albumin.
　　f. Portal systemic shunt.
　　g. Careful monitoring of the status of the patient regarding metabolic condition, fluid, and electrolytes.
　　h. Mechanical ventilation may be needed.

Chapter 5

Renal Diseases

Acute Renal Failure

Acute renal failure is characterized by sudden rapid decline or cessation in renal function limiting the ability of the kidney to maintain a normal chemical environment. As a result, there are progressive azotemia and increase of serum creatinine and usually decreased urine output. There may be anuria (urine less than 50 ml/day), oliguria (urine less than 400 ml/day) or even polyuria (urine more than 1800 ml/day). Oliguria is better defined as urine production at a rate below 0.5 ml/kg/hr.

Predisposing Factors

1. History of diabetes mellitus, hypertension, and gout or renal failure.
2. Use of nephrotoxic drugs like aminoglycosides.
3. Massive trauma, crush injury, and severe allergic reactions.

Causes

1. **Prerenal**: Severe shock, hypotension, hypovolemia, hypoxia, mismatched blood transfusion, DIC, jaundice, cirrhosis of liver, extensive trauma, burns,

pancreatitis, septicemia, endotoxemia, severe hypertension, etc.
2. **Renal**: Acute glomerulonephritis, severe pyelonephritis, nephrotoxic drugs like heavy metals, carbon tetrachloride, sulfonamides, and ethylene glycol.
3. **Postrenal**:
   a. Mechanical obstruction involving ureters and urethra: Calculi, blood clots, tumors, and prostatic hypertrophy.
   b. Functional obstruction: Diabetic neuropathy, pregnancy, and spinal cord diseases.

Acute renal failure is subdivided in four stages:
1. Initiation stage
2. Established stage
3. Diuretic stage
4. Recovery stage.

Diagnosis

1. **History and physical examination**: Hereditary diseases, any exposure to toxin, past kidney disease, and urine volume measurement. Bladder catheterization to exclude lower tract obstruction.
2. **Urine analysis**: Color, casts, sediments, presence of red blood cell, uric acid crystals, urine electrolytes, creatinine, osmolality, urine pH, and specific gravity.
3. **Electrolyte estimation**: Serum, sodium, potassium, chloride, phosphate, calcium, magnesium, and creatinine.
4. Blood urea nitrogen, serum and urine creatinine. BUN: serum creatinine ratios in excess of 15 may indicate a prerenal cause.
   a. Urine plasma creatinine ratio more than 20 indicates prerenal azotemia, less than 20 is acute renal failure.

b. Urine sodium concentration less than 20 indicates prerenalazotemia, more than 40 is acute renal failure.
c. Urine/plasma osmolality more than 1.2 in prerenal azotemia, less than 1.2 in acute renal failure.
d. Fractional excretion of sodium is calculated as:

$$\frac{\text{Urine/plasma sodium}}{\text{Urine/plasma creatinine}} \times 100$$

It is less than 1 in prerenal azotemia and more than 2 in acute renal failure.

5. **Monitoring of hemodynamics**: Assessment of intravascular volume, monitoring of CVP, and pulmonary artery occlusive pressure.
6. Renal ultrasound.
7. Renal scan.
8. Arterial blood gas analysis.
9. **Fluid challenge test**: A bolus of 200–500 ml is given IV followed by loop or osmotic diuretic. If urine output does not increase to 30–40 ml/hr over next hour helps to confirm acute renal failure.

Clinical Manifestations

1. Initially, there is an oliguric phase at the period of tubular necrosis and later it is followed by diuretic phase at the time of epithelial regeneration.
2. Pain in the loin, cloudy or bloody urine, edema, polydipsia, and disturbance in vision or hearing.
3. History of hypertension, nephrotoxic drugs, exposure of chemicals, heavy metals. Recent history of major trauma, infection, allergy, etc.
4. Weakness, confusion, and edema.
5. Rapid, regular deep respiratory rate.
6. Tachycardia, hypertension, and arrhythmia.
7. Pulmonary edema.

Management

1. Hypotension should be carefully assessed and treated with IV infusion of saline and vasopressors. Volume replacement may help to treat prerenal azotemia. Volume overload in an oliguric patient needs dialysis.
2. Metabolic acidosis should be corrected with sodium bicarbonate. Underlying cause of severe metabolic acidosis should be detected.
3. Hyperkalemia needs correction and in extreme cases dialysis is indicated.
4. Obstructive uropathy needs early correction.
5. Dialysis is most important in management of acute renal failure. Monitoring of serum electrolytes, BUN and creatinine, calcium, and phosphate levels are mandatory at frequent intervals.
6. Fluid and electrolyte management is vital and should be done with sensible precautions.
7. Diet should provide adequate calorie to prevent catabolism. Sodium, potassium, protein, and phosphate should be judiciously given.
8. Serum calcium and phosphate should be maintained near normal levels. Hypocalcemic tetany or cardiac arrhythmias need treatment with IV calcium gluconate.
9. Uric acid level needs monitoring. Higher level needs correction with allopurinol, otherwise urate nephropathy may occur.
10. In acute renal failure, dialysis is usually indicated in cases:
    a. Volume overload
    b. Severe hyperkalemia
    c. Severe electrolyte disturbances
    d. Severe metabolic acidosis
    e. Uremic
    f. Uremic pericarditis.

It is also indicated in cases of excessive catabolism and where there is need for aggressive protein and calorie supplementation.
11. Following the course of dialysis dietary management needs adequate consideration. It relaxes the restriction of protein, fluid, and salt intake. Protein intake 1–2 gm/kg or more may be allowed. Intravenous infusion of essential amino acids may be helpful to prevent catabolism. Fluid and electrolyte supplements should depend on patient's weight, activity, and serum electrolyte levels.
12. In the recovery phase, a progressive increase in urinary output occurs. Fluid replacement needs extra care and should be guided by urinary volume measurement, determination of daily weight, and measurement of urine electrolyte levels. Continued improvement of renal function is expected.

Complications

1. Infection is most common. Prevention should always be tried. Minimum catheterization. Antibiotic therapy—Antibiotic doses should be adjusted according to level of renal function.
2. Hypertension: Diuresis, dialysis, antihypertensive drugs—Clonidine, prazocin, vasodilators. Hypertensive crisis may be tackled with IV sodium nitroprusside.
3. Electrolytes should always be monitored. Hyponatremia and hyperkalemia should be carefully treated.
4. Gastrointestinal bleeding may occur and it also needs supportive treatment.
5. Anemia may occur and usually normocytic normochromic type. Blood transfusion may be needed.

6. Neurologic complications: Lethargy, mental changes, convulsion, etc. are common. These need full evaluation and early treatment. Neuropathy and myoclonic twitching are indications of early dialysis.
7. Uremic pericarditis, pericardial tamponade needs early detection and prompt management.

Chronic Renal Failure

Chronic renal failure involves a significant reduction in the glomerular filtration rate mostly from many chronic progressive renal diseases resulting in functioning nephron loss. Ultimately, it causes an irreversible loss of renal function and requires treatment with dialysis or kidney transplantation for survival.

Predisposing Factors

1. Past history of acute nephritis, nephrotic syndrome, urinary obstruction, hematuria, proteinurea, abuse of antibiotics, analgesics, and nephrotoxic drugs.
2. Present history of diabetes mellitus, hypertension, and cardiovascular disease.
3. Family history of polycystic renal disease, sickle cell disease, gout, renal calculi, etc.

Causes

1. Chronic destructive renal diseases:
    a. Chronic glomerulonephritis.
    b. Periarteritis nodosa.
    c. Rheumatoid arthritis.
    d. Systemic lupus erythematosus.
2. Infection: Pyelonephritis.
3. Chronic urinary tract obstruction: Prostatic enlargement.
4. Chronic renal vascular disease:

a. Malignant hypertension: Hypertensive glomerulosclerosis
   b. Gout
   c. Diabetes mellitus: Diabetic nephropathy
   d. Renal vein thrombosis.
5. Congenital: Polycystic disease.
   - Common causes of rapid worsening of chronic renal failure:
     a. Hypertension/hypotension
     b. Infection
     c. Volume depletion and dehydration
     d. Nephrotoxic agents/drugs
     e. Severe congestive heart failure.

Clinical Manifestations

1. Inability to control water excretion.
2. Fluid overload/edema, pulmonary edema, and cerebral edema.
3. Chronic renal failure may have three stages:
   a. Decreased renal reserve. GFR within 50–80 ml/min (Normal 125 ml/min).
   b. In renal insufficiency, GFR 12–50 ml/min Nocturia. BUN increased, serum creatinine increased.
   c. In established renal failure, GFR less than 12 ml/min. Uremia, anemia, hyperkalemia, BUN increased. Serum creatinine increased, bleeding time increased. Loss of more than 90% of functioning nephrons results in uremia and the need for dialysis.
4. Metabolic acidosis, Kussmaul type of respiration.
5. Hypocalcemia, phosphate retention, failure to activate vitamin D leading to cramps, tetany, and convulsions.
6. Chronic anemia, resistant type due to depression of bone marrow, deficient erythropoietin, reduced RBC survival. Oxyhemoglobin dissociation curve shifted to left.

7. Anorexia, nausea/vomiting, hiccup, and aspiration.
8. Hematemesis, melena, and diarrhea.
9. Headache, lassitude, malaise, tremor, insomnia, mental depression, confusion, and uremic coma.
10. Malignant hypertension and its complications.
11. Pericarditis with or without effusion and cardiac tamponade.
12. Coagulopathy and DIC.
13. Skin pigmentation, purpura, and pruritis.
14. Immunity depressed.
15. Chest X-ray: Uremic lung.
16. Renal ultrasound.
17. Renal biopsy.

Biochemical Features of Chronic Renal Failure

1. Impaired water metabolism: Water overload.
2. Sodium retention.
3. Potassium retention and hyperkalemia.
4. Acidosis.
5. Retention of phosphate and low calcium level.
6. Retention of urea, uric acid, amines, creatinine, etc.
7. Magnesium metabolism and excretion altered.
8. Urine: Osmolality decreased, pH increased, presence of RBC, casts, epithelial cells, and protein. Specific gravity increased/decreased. Urine creatinine clearance—Decreased.
9. Arterial blood gas studies: Decreased pH and HCO_3.

Management

1. Remaining kidney function should be preserved:
   a. Avoid dehydration and hypotension.
   b. Avoid infection and nephrotoxic drugs.
   c. Prevent obstruction to flow of urine.

2. Try to delay development of uremic syndrome:
   a. Protein restriction
   b. Maintain anabolic state
   c. Restriction of fluids.
3. Maintain fluid and electrolyte balance and acid-base balance.
4. Nutrition should be adequate.
5. Drug therapy:
   a. Diuretics: Use of diuretics is controversial. It can be used with extreme caution when the kidneys are still making urine.
   b. Antihypertensive drugs to treat hypertension. Dialysis can also control hypertension.
   c. Adrenergic blocking drugs: In severe hypotension and shock, adequate fluid therapy is indicated. Phentolamine or phenoxybenzamine may be used as it may increase the urine output.
   d. Hyperkalemia should be treated with adequate IV glucose and insulin. Calcium gluconate is also indicated to antagonise the effects of hyperkalemia. Dialysis may be needed in extreme cases.
   e. Maintenance of nutrition. Low protein diet.
   f. Anemia: Iron and folic acid. Blood transfusion may be needed in resistant cases.
   g. Electrolyte and acid-base balance.
   h. Infection: Antibiotics, nephrotoxic drugs should be avoided.
   i. Heart failure needs adequate treatment. It may increase renal perfusion and enhance renal function.
   j. Acidosis: Sodium bicarbonate.
   k. Hyperuricemia: Allopurinol.
   l. Constipation: Stool softeners and laxatives.
   m. Calcium replacement.

n. Vitamins, iron, and folic acid.
o. Blood transfusion and packed RBC.
p. Indications for dialysis in chronic renal failure:
  i. Volume overload
  ii. Hyperkalemia
  iii. Severe electrolyte disturbances
  iv. Severe acidosis
  v. Uremic manifestations
  vi. Excessive catabolism
  vii. Uremic pericarditis.

Hemodialysis

It is a very reliable lifesaving procedure. It needs an arteriovenous fistula for better hemodialysis. Here, arterial blood is taken out of the patient and passed through one side of a colloid membrane and then after dialysis, the blood is returned IV. The membrane is permeable to water, electrolytes, and glucose, but not to protein and red blood cells. By suitable adjustments of dialysis fluid, the water, electrolyte, and acid-base balance are maintained.

- Hemodialysis may have some complications:
  a. Membrane leakage.
  b. Air bubbles.
  c. Dialysis-related pericarditis.
  d. Dialysis disequilibrium syndrome and convulsion cramps, and mental changes.
  e. Dialysis hypotension.
  f. Vascular access complications: Infection, arteriovenous fistula, and thrombosis.

Ultrafiltration

It is the method of removing volume without altering the chemical nature of plasma. It can be done during dialysis by manipulating transmembrane pressures or it can be performed independently.

Peritoneal Dialysis

Here, the peritoneal cavity and its vessels act as dialysis membrane. Glucose in dialysate provides an adjustable osmotic gradient for ultrafiltration. The technique is simple and needs simple apparatus. The procedure essentially consists of passing a catheter through the abdominal wall below umbilicus into the peritoneal cavity, kept preferably in the rectovesical pouch. Here, the urea, hydrogen ions, electrolytes and other waste products can pass into the dialysate and this can be taken out from the abdominal cavity.

- Dialysate may vary according to the clinical condition of the patient. Usually, it contains sodium 141 mEq/L, chloride 101 mEq/L, calcium 3.5 mEq/L, lactate 45 mEq/L, bisulfate 1 mEq/L, and dextrose 1.5%. But in cases with water retention, the dialyzing fluid should contain dextrose 7%, while other ingredients remain same. Usually, one liter of solution is passed into the peritoneal cavity within 10–20 minutes and then kept for some 20 minutes before draining off. Usually, the cycle takes about one hour.

Complications of peritoneal dialysis—
1. Failure of drainage—Fluid retention and heart failure
2. Hyperglycemia
3. Protein loss
4. Electrolyte abnormalities
5. Peritonitis and perforation of viscera
6. Infection
7. Cardiopulmonary embarassment.

Renal Transplantation

It is indicated in some selected patients suffering from end-stage renal disease mostly due to diabetes and hypertension. These patients are usually getting hemodialysis for a long time.

Some Nephrotoxic Drugs

A. Antibiotics: Sulfonamides (sulfamethoxazole), amphotericin B, aminoglycosides (kanamycin, gentamicin, tobramycin, etc.) cephalosporins, etc.
B. Diuretics: Osmotic agents like sucrose, mannitol, dextran loop diuretics (frusemide and ethacrynic acid)
C. Analgesics: Aspirin and phenacetin
D. Anesthetics: Methoxyflurane, halothane, cyclopropane, etc.
E. Others: Iodinated contrast media, ethylene glycol, methanol, intravenous acyclovir, and cisplatin.

Diabetic Nephropathy

Long-standing diabetes mellitus can cause significant renal damage. Here the glomerular filtration increases initially, returns to normal with further damage of the kidney and then continues to fall. Massive proteinurea occurs. Diabetic retinopathy may also be present in such cases. On ultrasound, kidneys are either normal or enlarged. Biopsy usually shows diffuse or nodular intercapillary glomerulosclerosis.

Management

1. Control blood sugar.
2. Control blood pressure.

3. ACE inhibition or angiotensin H. receptor blockade can reduce hyperfiltration and proteinurea.
4. General supportive care.
5. Treat anemia, acidosis, and elevated phosphorus.
6. Protein restriction may be done.
7. Renal transplant in selected extreme cases.

Chapter 6

Endocrine Dysfunctions

Thyroid Storm/Thyrotoxic Crisis

Thyroid storm or thyrotoxic crisis is an exacerbation in intensity of the features of thyrotoxicosis. This life-threatening metabolic crisis is usually precipitated by surgery, particularly in patients who have not been treated adequately in preoperative period. It is characterized by hyperthermia, severe tachycardia, tachypnea, and an altered mental state.

Patients at Risk

1. Poorly controlled thyrotoxicosis.
2. Following radioactive iodine therapy.
3. Excessive administration of exogenous thyroid hormone.

Predisposing Factors

1. Surgery, thyroid or nonthyroid.
2. Infection.
3. Severe emotional upset.
4. Diabetic ketoacidosis.
5. Congestive heart failure and myocardial infarction.
6. Burns and trauma.

7. Toxemia, pregnancy, and childbirth.
8. Iodine containing X-ray contrast.

Pathophysiology

1. Sudden increase in circulating thyroid hormones.
2. Exhaustion of the body to circulating thyroxines.
3. Relative adrenal insufficiency.

Clinical Features

1. High fever.
2. Increased metabolic rate of the body, increased carbohydrate and fat metabolism.
3. Increased heart rate, atrial fibrillation, and heart failure.
4. Increased rate and depth of respiration.
5. Sweating, dehydration, shock, and electrolyte imbalance hypotension.
6. Confusion, delirium, agitation, stupor, and coma.

Laboratory Investigations

1. Serum T_3 and T_3 by radioimmune assay
2. Plasma cortisol
3. Serum electrolytes
4. Blood sugar estimation
5. Complete blood count
6. ECG and tachyarrhythmias
7. Radioiodine uptake scan
8. Serum creatine phosphokinase to exclude malignant hyperthermia.

Management

Preventive measures

1. Operation should be done in euthyroid state.

2. Hyperthyroidism should always be treated adequately.
3. β-blocker drugs may be helpful in pre and postoperative period.
4. Operation should be delayed if resting pulse rate is more than 90 beats per minute.
5. Intercurrent infection and heart failure should be adequately treated in preoperative period.

Treatment

1. Restoration and maintenance of vital functions:
   a. Fluids and electrolytes.
   b. Vasopressors.
   c. IV infusion and glucose.
   d. Oxygen therapy.
2. Control of hyperpyrexia:
   a. Tepid sponging, cooling fans, cooling blanket, and gastric lavage with ice-cold saline.
   b. Promote reduction of body temperature.
   c. Monitoring of body temperature is essential.
3. Antithyroid drugs to block further thyroid hormone synthesis and release:
   a. Sodium iodide.
   b. Carbimazole.
4. Hydrocortisone and dexamethasone to correct the relative adrenocortical insufficiency.
5. Correction of sympathetic overactivity—Propranolol, reserpine and esmolol.
6. Digitalis, inotropes, diuretics, and IPPV—It may be needed to manage cardiac failure.
7. Precipitating factors should be identified and treated.
8. Effectiveness of therapy should always be monitored.

Myxedema Coma

It is a life-threatening clinical condition with severe thyroid failure. Severe and long-standing low-levels of thyroid hormone produce an extreme state of hypometabolism. It is characterized by hypothermia, an altered mental state, and ultimately coma.

Causes

1. Patients suffering from primary hypothyroidism.
2. Predisposing factors:
   a. Narcotics, tranquilizers, and anesthetic drugs
   b. Exposure to cold
   c. Infection
   d. Trauma
   e. Surgery
   f. Cerebrovascular accident
   g. Congestive cardiac failure
   h. Hypothermia
   i. Hypoglycemia
   j. Hypercapnic narcosis.

Pathophysiology

1. Lack of thyroid hormone in the body.
2. Decreased metabolic rate.
3. Decreased heat production.
4. Decreased carbohydrate and fat metabolism.
5. Decreased cardiac activity.
6. Decreased respiratory activity.
7. Decreased mental status.
8. Decreased muscle tone and reactivity.

Clinical Manifestations

1. Myxedema—Nonpitting edema of subcutaneous tissues.
2. Unresponsiveness and coma.
3. Hypothermia—Levels below 30°C carry grave risk.

4. Hypotension
5. Hypoventilation
6. Bradycardia
7. Hyponatremia.

Investigations

1. Serum thyroxine—Decreased.
2. Serum T_3—Decreased.
3. TSH—Increased.
4. Arterial blood gas analysis—Decreased PaO_2 and increased $PaCO_2$.
5. Blood sugar may be increased.
6. Complete blood count.
7. Serum cholesterol, and creatinine may be increased.
8. Chest X-ray—Enlarged heart shadow.
9. ECG—Low voltage ECG.
10. Echocardiogram.

Management

1. Supportive therapy:
   a. Hypoventilation: Adequate oxygenation and ventilation.
   b. Hypotension: Pressor agents and IV fluids.
   c. Hypothermia: Thyroxine therapy—Treatment with external heat may worsen the condition.
   d. Hyponatremia: Thyroxine therapy—Injudicious fluid restriction.
   e. Hypoglycemia: Glucose solution infusion.
   f. Maintain fluid and electrolyte balance.
   g. Monitoring of vital functions at regular intervals.
2. Drug therapy:
   a. Thyroid hormone: Levothyroxine 200–500 µg IV.
   b. Glucocorticoids: Hydrocortisone.
3. Treatment of precipitating factors.

Diabetic Ketoacidosis

Diabetic ketoacidosis is an acute metabolic disorder due to lack of insulin resulting in a significant elevation of blood sugar and increased levels of ketoacids such as acetoacetate and β-hydroxy butyric acid in the blood and urine in diabetic patients.

Causes

An absolute or relative insulin-deficiency causing mobilization and oxidation of fatty acids with production of ketoacids.
1. It is a complication of diabetes mellitus and mostly in insulin-dependent type of diabetic patients.
2. Undiagnosed or inadequately controlled diabetic patients.
3. Predisposing factors:
   a. Infection.
   b. Nausea/vomiting and diarrhea.
   c. Trauma, injury and surgery. Increased catabolic stress.
   d. Pregnancy.
   e. Insufficient coverage of insulin.
   f. Some drugs may affect glucose-insulin balance such as steroids, catecholamines, phenothiazines, aspirin, indomethacin, etc.

Pathophysiology

1. There is insufficient amount of insulin to tackle the amount of glucose.
2. Increased blood glucose.
3. Increased ketogenesis, increased production of ketone bodies.
4. Serum osmolality changes lead to intracellular and extracellular dehydration.

5. Renal excretion of glucose increased.
6. Increased production of acids and metabolic acidosis.
7. Tissue hypoxia, anaerobic glycolysis and production of lactate.

Clinical Manifestations

Polyuria, polydipsia, polyphagia, nausea/vomiting, epigastric discomfort, abdominal cramp/pain, weakness, weight loss and drowsiness.

Lethargy, tachycardia, hypotension, tachypnea, acetone/sweet odor to breath, hot dry skin, dry mucous membrane, dehydration, confusion and coma.

Laboratory

1. Blood glucose level increased.
2. Urine glucose increased.
3. Urine analysis—Acetone present—Ketonuria.
4. Serum electrolytes—Hyponatremia and hypokalemia.
5. Serum osmolality widely increased.
6. Arterial blood gases—Arterial pH less than 7.3, bicarbonate less than 9 mmol/L—Metabolic acidosis.
7. Serum creatinine level increased.
8. Blood urea nitrogen level increased.
9. Estimation of serum ketone bodies—Increased.

Management

1. Adequate oxygenation and ventilation.
2. Adequate fluid management. Correction of dehydration.
3. IV infusion with normal saline.
4. Soluble insulin 20 units IV and then IV infusion 10 units per hour. Very low-dose of insulin 6–8 units per hour by continuous infusion is helpful. Control of blood sugar is most important.

5. Potassium replacement.
6. Sodium bicarbonate may be needed to treat metabolic acidosis. Dose should be determined by blood gas analysis.
7. Identify and treat precipitating factors.
8. Prevent complications.
9. Monitor the vital signs and blood glucose, electrolytes and arterial blood gas studies frequently.
10. Monitor urinary output, electrocardiogram and serum potassium to assess renal and cardiac function.

Complications

- Cerebral edema: It may be due to over-rapid correction of hyperosmolality, the use of excessive alkali and too rapid lowering of the blood sugar.
- Renal failure: It may be due to prolonged period of shock and hypovolemia and delayed treatment.
- Cardiac failure: Particularly in elderly patients when large quantities of intravenous fluids are given.
- Disseminated intravascular coagulopathy can also occur.
- Pulmonary edema.
- Electrolyte imbalance.

Hyperglycemic Hyperosmolar Nonketotic Coma

It is an acute complication of diabetes mellitus where there is insulin resistance and a relative insulin-deficiency resulting in severe hyperglycemia, hyperosmolality with osmotic diuresis and mild or absent ketonemia.

Causes

1. Previously undiagnosed diabetes mellitus (usually noninsulin-dependent cases).

2. Middle-aged/elderly individuals.
3. Obesity.
4. Predisposing factors:
   a. Acute illness (infection, burns, pancreatitis, myocardial infarction and cerebrovascular accident).
   b. Trauma, surgery, and stress.
   c. Hypothermia.
   d. Drugs like propranolol, phenytoin, frusemide, thiazide diuretics, and steroids.
   e. Peritoneal dialysis with hypertonic glucose dialysate solutions.
   f. Total parenteral nutrition solution, high-calorie enteric feeding solutions.
   g. Hemodialysis.

Pathophysiology

1. Predisposing factors precipitate the release of hormones such as glucagon, cortisol, and adrenaline. All these increase blood sugar.
2. Insulin resistance and relative insulin-deficiency are present.
3. Severe hyperglycemia causes cellular dehydration and an osmotic diuresis and large amounts of water and electrolytes are depleted.
4. Hypovolemia and hyperosmolality develop.
5. Thus the clinical effects include severe hyperglycemia, hyperosmolality, severe dehydration, and electrolyte imbalance.

Clinical Features

1. Polyuria, polydipsia, and polyphagia
2. Weight loss, weakness, and mental fatigue
3. Headache, stupor, comatose, and coma
4. Convulsion

5. Paresis
6. Tachycardia, hypotension, and shock
7. Severe dehydration
8. Renal failure.

Laboratory Findings

1. Blood sugar elevated > 600 mg%.
2. Serum osmolality > 330 mOsm/L.
3. Serum sodium and potassium may be normal, decreased or increased.
4. Arterial blood gas analysis: Normal or mild acidosis. Bicarbonate normal or only slightly reduced.
5. Serum ketones: Absence of significant ketonemia.
6. Urine analysis: Glucose present, increased specific gravity, and normal or mild increase in ketones.

Management

1. Precipitating factors should be detected.
2. Adequate oxygenation and ventilation. Nasogastric tube may be helpful to prevent aspiration pneumonitis.
3. Intravenous infusion to correct volume deficit. Isotonic normal saline is preferred. Serum sodium or osmolality measurements should guide the fluid therapy. Care should be taken in aged patients and in patients with myocardial infarction, heart failure or renal failure. Frequent assessment and invasive hemodynamic monitoring are essential.
4. Bicarbonate therapy to combat lactic acidosis. Phosphate should be monitored and may have to be replaced.
5. Potassium replacement may be needed in presence of hypokalemia. Potassium should be administered only after insulin has begun to act, otherwise severe hyperkalemia may occur.

6. Insulin treatment is necessary to restore glucose homeostasis. But blood glucose level should guide the therapy. Oral hypoglycemic drugs should be avoided in such cases.
7. Monitoring of therapy is essential. Blood glucose and serum electrolytes should be assessed at frequent intervals.
8. Thrombotic episodes may occur and this is mostly due to intense dehydration and other factors. Anticoagulant therapy may be indicated in such cases.

Hypoglycemia

Hypoglycemia may occur as a complication of therapy with oral hypoglycemic agents and with insulin. It is less common in nondiabetic individuals. It is life-threatening and needs prompt treatment and correction of the underlying causes. A blood glucose level of less than 70 mg% manifests the features of hypoglycemia.

Causes

1. Change in timing of meals or content of meals.
2. Overdose of oral hypoglycemic drugs or insulin.
3. Increase in physical activities.

Clinical Manifestations

1. Irritability, restlessness, headache, diaphoresis, tachycardia, and confusion.
2. Convulsion, stupor, and coma.
3. Tachycardia, hypertension, and cardiac arrhythmias may occur and these are all catecholamine related.
4. Blood glucose level less than 70 mg% constitutes hypoglycemia.
5. Hypoglycemic manifestations may be masked by general anesthesia and β-blockers.

Management

1. Oral carbohydrate in mild cases.
2. IV glucose solution—50 ml of 50% glucose solution initially and then 5–10% glucose solution infusion. Blood glucose level should be kept at about 150 mg%.
3. Glucagon IM or subcutaneous may also be tried.
4. For prevention, drug therapy should be adjusted as dictated by blood glucose estimations and urine analysis. Diet and physical activity also need sensible adjustments.
5. The patient should bear an identification card for safety. The patient should be advised to carry some carbohydrate and take immediately when he feels discomfort and restlessness.
6. Spontaneous hypoglycemia may occur in nondiabetic patients, but it is not so common. Hypoglycemia may occur on prolonged fasting. A normal subject is able to maintain blood glucose level with 72 hours of fasting. The other causes may include insulinoma, alcohol intoxication, severe liver disease, chronic renal failure, hypothyroidism, adrenocortical insufficiency, etc. Thus, management should be according to the cause.
7. Reactive hypoglycemia may occur in postprandial period from the action of insulin secreted in response to meals. It may also occur following partial gastrectomy. A change in eating habits and/or food content may be helpful in such cases.
8. Treatment of hypoglycemia should be started even when it is suspected as therapy for hypoglycemia carries little risk, but waiting for clinical laboratory results or failure to treat hypoglycemia may be dangerous.

Complications

1. Central nervous system injury
2. Cardiac arrest.

Acute Adrenocortical Insufficiency

Acute adrenocortical insufficiency often designated acute adrenal crisis is a serious life-threatening condition that is characterized by an absence or deficiency of glucocorticoids and mineralocorticoids. It is also known as addisonian crisis.

Predisposing Factors

1. These patients of primary adrenocortical insufficiency are lacking sufficient cortisol and aldosterone.
2. Some factors may be responsible for acute crisis and these may include acute infection, trauma, surgery, myocardial infarction, etc. Thromboembolic disorders, coagulopathies, septicemia, etc. may also increase the risk.
3. Some drugs like aminoglutethimide, ketoconazole, phenytoin, rifampin, etc. can inhibit steroid synthesis or enhance steroid metabolism in patients with deficient adrenocortical reserve.

Pathophysiology

1. Deficient mineralocorticoid activity: Lack of aldosterone causes loss of sodium and water in urine, decreased extracellular fluid volume, hyperkalemia, and acidosis.
2. Deficient glucocorticoid activity: Hypoglycemia, hypotension, and inability to tolerate stress.

Clinical Manifestations

1. Anorexia, nausea/vomiting, fatigue, weakness, headache, and thirst.

2. Dry mucous membrane, oliguria, tachycardia, hypotension, fever, confusion, acute abdominal pain, and coma.
3. Laboratory findings:
   a. Serum electrolytes—Hyponatremia and hyperkalemia.
   b. Blood glucose level—Hypoglycemia.
4. Blood gas analysis: Metabolic acidosis.
5. Plasma cortisol level decreased.

Management

1. Effective management needs prompt recognition and treatment with IV fluids and glucocorticoids is mandatory. One should not wait for laboratory confirmation.
2. Rapid IV fluid administration for volume repletion. Electrolyte balance should also be ensured. Hemodynamic support with vasopressors or inotropes.
3. Glucocorticoid therapy: IV hydrocortisone or its equivalent. It should not be discontinued abruptly. Dose may be governed by the severity of the precipitating cause.
4. Mineralocorticoid therapy is not required immediately, but water and salt replacement is essential.
5. Monitoring of plasma cortisol level is always helpful.
6. Precipitating factors should be sought and judged.
7. Intensive supportive care:
   a. Fluid and electrolyte balance
   b. IV glucose to treat hypoglycemia
   c. Hyperthermia should be tackled
   d. Promote adequate oxygenation and tissue perfusion
   e. Ensure hemodynamic stability
8. Complications:
   a. Cardiac arrest.
   b. Complications of steroid therapy.

Chapter 7

Temperature Illness

Heat Stroke

It is a life-threatening heat illness resulting from excessive body temperature. It is mostly due to overloading or derangement of the heat dissipating mechanisms of the body. It is a serious condition with high morbidity and mortality rate and these are mostly related to the degree and duration of the hyperpyrexia.

Clinical Features

1. Hyperpyrexia: The core temperature may exceed 105°F.
2. Central nervous system dysfunction: Delirium, psychosis, convulsion, and coma.
3. Anhidrosis is common. Sweating may be seen in some cases particularly in exertional heat stroke of rapid onset.
4. Hypotension, rapid pulse, circulatory collapse due to hypovolemia, and cardiac dysfunction.
5. Serum enzymes are elevated due to cellular damage.
6. Acid-base and electrolytes alter, and dehydration, metabolic acidosis.
7. Coagulation dysfunction.
8. Hypoxemia and cellular hypoxia in different organs.

Complications

1. Aspiration and bronchopneumonia
2. Cardiac arrhythmias, and cardiac failure
3. Hepatic failure
4. Renal failure and myoglobinuria
5. Neurological deficits
6. Bleeding diathesis.

All these complications are mostly due to dysfunction or failure of any body system resulting from direct excessive body temperature and cellular damage.

Management

1. The primary aim is to reduce body temperature towards near normal and to support vital functions of the body.
2. Cooling may be tried with ice-water or ice-sponging. Aircoolers and electric fans may be used. Shivering should be prevented with the help of chlorpromazine. Active cooling should be discontinued when the core temperature reaches 102°F, otherwise hypothermia may occur.
3. Adequate oxygenation.
4. Intravenous fluids.
5. Sodium bicarbonate IV to combat metabolic acidosis.
6. Mannitol may be helpful to treat oliguria.
7. Fresh whole blood, fresh frozen plasma, platelets, etc. may be needed to treat bleeding diatheses.
8. Monitoring of body temperature is needed at regular short intervals.

Malignant Hyperthermia

It is a clinical syndrome of highly accelerated metabolic state often characterized by hyperpyrexia, tachycardia, tachypnea, cyanosis, hypoxemia, and death. It occurs in susceptible patients when triggered by some agent such as halothane and succinylcholine. It may occur in all individuals both male and female and in all ages, but the incidence is rare below the age of 3 years and in geriatric patients.

- It is an inherited neuromuscular disorder (autosomal dominant, familial). The gene for malignant hyperthermia is also the genetic coding site for the calcium release channel of skeletal muscle sarcoplasmic reticulum. A defect in this channel causes sustained higher concentrations of calcium in the myoplasm resulting in persistent skeletal muscle contracture when susceptible patients are exposed to triggering agents. This is associated with all signs of hypermetabolism such as tachycardia, arterial hypoxemia, metabolic acidosis, respiratory acidosis, and profound hyperpyrexia.

However, the syndrome may be either rigid or nonrigid type, depending on the presence or absence of muscle contractures respectively.

Clinical Features

1. Fulminant pyrexia—Sustained rise to as high as 42°C or more.
2. Tachycardia, tachypnea, hypoxemia, hypercapnia, sweating, and cyanosis.
3. Hypotension.
4. Metabolic and respiratory acidosis.
5. Oliguria, acute renal failure, and myoglobinurea.
6. Hypertonicity of muscles. May affect whole body.
7. Hyperkalemia and hypocalcemia.
8. Convulsion.
9. Cardiac failure.
10. DIC may occur.

Laboratory Findings

1. Blood gas analysis: Low pH, low PaO_2, increased $PaCO_2$. Check O_2 saturation and end-tidal CO_2.
2. Electrolyte estimation: Increased serum potassium, calcium and magnesium, and low serum sodium.
3. Serum lactate, pyruvate, CPK, LDH, aldolase and magnesium increased, serum SGOT and SGPT increased.
4. Total blood count.
5. Urine analysis: Myoglobinurea occurs late.
6. Electrocardiogram: Dysrhythmia—Peaked T-wave is an early sign of hyperkalemia.
7. Coagulation studies.
8. Check core temperature at short intervals.

Diagnosis/Identification of Susceptible Patients

1. Past anesthetic history may often be helpful. Detailed history of any anesthetic death or difficulty in the family.
2. Myopathic syndromes may often be associated.
3. Elevation of plasma CPK level is mostly evident.
4. Skeletal muscle biopsy (vastus muscle of thigh) subjected to in vitro isometric contracture testing in presence of caffeine and/or halothane gives the definitive test of susceptibility to malignant hyperthermia.

Management

1. All inhalation agents and triggering agents like halothane should be stopped. Surgery should be concluded as early as possible. Known triggering agents are all inhalational anesthetics except nitrous oxide and depolarising muscle relaxants.

2. Adequate oxygenation with 100% oxygen.
3. Dantrolene 2.5 mg/kg IV initially followed by repeat doses every 5–10 minutes until symptoms are controlled. The total dose should not exceed 10 mg/kg. Dantrolene is lifesaving.
4. Active cooling: Ice-cold saline IV, gastric or peritoneal lavage with ice-cold saline. Ice-sponging, ice-cold blanket, etc. Cooling should be stopped when core temperature reaches 38°C.
5. Adequate hydration. Fluid input-output chart.
6. Sodium bicarbonate to combat metabolic acidosis.
7. IV lignocaine or procainamide to treat ventricular arrhythmias.
8. Maintain urinary output. Frusemide or mannitol may be helpful.
9. General supportive measures. Maintain fluid and electrolyte balance. Correct hyperkalemia with frusemide or IV glucose and insulin.
10. Careful monitoring of vital signs is essential.
11. Common complications include acute renal failure, pulmonary edema, cardiac failure, consumption coagulopathy, neurological sequelae, etc. These should be tackled, whenever needed.
12. The patient should be warned against the serious nature of the syndrome and should carry an identification card. Family members also need investigation for susceptibility to malignant hyperthermia.

Hypothermia

Hypothermia is a clinical condition where the internal (core) body temperature is less than 35°C (95°F). It is mostly due to exposure to cold environment. It is most common in neonates, young children, and elderly persons whose thermoregulatory mechanism are either immature or impaired. Hypothermia is often graded as mild (32°C–35°C) moderate (28°C–32°C) and severe (less than 32°C).

Predisposing Factors

1. Malnutrition: Exposure to low ambient temperature.
2. Alcohol/drug intoxication, overdose of barbiturates.
3. Metabolic disorders: Hyperglycemia, hypothyroidism, hypoadrenalism, and diabetic coma.
4. Central nervous system disorders, cerebrovascular accident, and high spinal cord injuries.
5. Severe sepsis.
6. Massive injuries and circulatory collapse.
7. Low environmental temperature and near drowning.
8. Prolonged anesthesia/surgery in air-conditioned theater particularly in neonates and infants.
9. Massive transfusion of cold refrigerated blood.

Pathophysiology/Manifestations

1. Following exposure in cold environment, there may be compensatory responses such as cutaneous vasodilation and shivering. Shivering usually does not occur when the core temperature is less than 32°C. Decreased metabolic rate.
2. Progressive decrease in respiratory minute volume, heart rate, cardiac output, and hypotension.
3. Hypovolemia resulting from intravascular fluid loss and cold diuresis.
4. Cardiac arrhythmias and conduction defects.
5. Central nervous system depression. Decreased level of consciousness.
6. Metabolic acidosis: Mild coagulopathies—Oxyhemoglobin dissociation curve shifts leftward.
7. Hyperglycemia/hypoglycemia.

8. ECG—Prolongation of PR, QRS, and QT intervals.
9. Profound hypothermia ultimately leads to death.

Complications

1. Cardiac arrhythmias and myocardial infarction.
2. Aspiration pneumonitis.
3. Pulmonary edema.
4. Acute pancreatitis.
5. Acute renal failure.
6. Intravascular thrombosis, abnormal blood coagulation, increased blood viscosity, and cerebrovascular accident.
7. Cardiac or respiratory arrest. Ventricular fibrillation.

Management

1. Careful monitoring of vital signs is essential. Maintain ambient temperature at 22°C or higher.
2. Intensive supportive care.
3. Heated humidified oxygenation is helpful, assisted ventilation.
4. Intravenous fluid therapy.
5. Rewarming:
   a. Passive rewarming: By insulating the patient from the environment with blankets is often helpful in mild degree of hypothermia.
   b. Active external rewarming: Application of heat to the surface of the body may also be tried.
   c. Active core rewarming: Application of exogenous heat to the body's core, radiant heaters, inhalation rewarming, heated and humidified inspired gases, heated peritoneal lavage. Extracorporeal blood rewarming may be needed in extreme cases.
6. Sodium bicarbonate IV to treat metabolic acidosis.
7. Hemodialysis or peritoneal dialysis with heated dialysate may also be indicated in certain cases.

8. Complications, if any, should be detected early and treated accordingly.
9. Hypothermia with cardiac arrest needs cardiopulmonary resuscitation and rapid core rewarming.
10. Hypothermic patients can tolerate prolonged CPR due to the protective effect of hypothermia on the central nervous system.
11. No patient should be declared dead while hypothermic.

Chapter 8

Poisoning

Self-poisoning

Self-poisoning is common in all countries. Mortality and morbidity rate are usually high. A few specific antidote is available and thus the physicians are to rely on the general principles of maintaining vital functions of the body and different methods to enhance the elimination of the drug. Specific or pharmacological antidotes, whenever known should need proper attention to tackle the cases.

Diagnosis

1. History of taking drugs and suicidal note.
2. History from a conscious patient, often very unreliable; any information from family and friends.
3. Drug bottles, ampoules, etc. if available.
4. Clinical features:
    a. Superficial blisters—Barbiturate poisoning.
    b. Venepuncture marks.
    c. Pupil size:
        i. Fixed dilated pupils: Diphenhydramine poisoning.
        ii. Pinpoint pupil: Opiate poisoning.
    d. Papilledema—Nalidixic acid.

e. Altered level of consciousness.
  f. Chest pain, any arrhythmia.
  g. Respiratory status and pulmonary edema.
  h. Nausea/vomiting, diarrhea, and abdominal pain.
5. a. Any tablet, bottle, and ampoule found with the patient.
  b. Unlabelled tablet may be sent to pharmacy.
  c. Blood and urine biochemistry. Gastric contents examination.
  d. But time should not be wasted for identification of the drug and treatment should be initiated immediately particularly to establish and maintain the vital functions of the body. However, blood report may be helpful in some cases such as salicylate poisoning and paracetamol poisoning, etc.
  e. Some diseases like meningitis, subarachnoid hemorrhage, head injury, and other causes of coma should always be excluded in the diagnosis of poisoning.
  f. Concomitant diseases such as cardiac, pulmonary, renal, hepatic, metabolic, and endocrinal dysfunction need appropriate evaluation as these may influence the prognosis.
  g. A knowledge of the drug pharmacology and toxic effects is essential to dictate the line of management.

Management

1. Maintenance of vital function and intensive supportive care are most important to manage poison cases.
   a. **Maintenance of ventilation**:
      i. Assessment of respiratory status: Physical examination, chest X-ray, and arterial blood gas studies.
      ii. Establish and maintain a clear patent airway and ventilation. Endotracheal intubation, IPPV. Adequate oxygenation.

b. **Maintenance of circulation**:
   i. Assessment of cardiovascular status, physical examination, ECG, and CVP monitoring.
   ii. Hypotension: Volume expansion, vasoactive drugs like dopamine, metaraminol, and noradrenaline.
   iii. Hypertension: It is not common, but hypertensive crisis may occur with sympathomimetic overdoses. Sodium nitroprusside, diazoxide, and β-blockers may be needed.
c. Antiarrhythmic drugs to treat arrhythmias.
d. Fluid and electrolyte balance.
e. **Central nervous system depression**:
   i. Care of the unconscious patient, supportive care.
   ii. Naloxone hydrochloride to reverse the depressant effects of opioid overdose.
f. **Convulsion**:
   i. Correction of metabolic and electrolyte disturbances.
   ii. Hypoxia and hypoglycemia should be corrected.
   iii. Drugs like diazepam, phenytoin, and phenobarbitone.
g. **Temperature illness**:
   i. Hyperthermia may occur in sympathomimetic or anticholinergic drug overdose. Maintenance of normothermia should be tried by all possible means, i.e. ice pack, ice-sponging, fans, coolers, etc.
   ii. Hypothermia: It is mostly due to sedative/hypnotic overdose. Gradual rewarming is beneficial.
h. **Metabolic acidosis**: It is common in intoxication with salicylates, methanol, etc. Sodium bicarbonate may be indicated.

2. Skin decontamination: Removal of clothing, washing with soda and water.
3. Prevention of drug absorption from gastrointestinal tract:

a. Induced emesis.
   b. Gastric lavage and irrigation.
   c. Activated charcoal.
   d. Catharsis: Laxative to speed the emptying of the poison from gastrointestinal tract.
4. Antidotes:
   a. Atropine sulfate and pralidoxime in organophosphorus poisoning.
   b. Naloxone in opioid poisoning.
5. Removal of absorbed drugs:
   a. Forced diuresis and/or hemoperfusion:
      i. Forced alkaline diuresis in salicylate, barbiturate poisoning. Mannitol or frusemide may be helpful.
      ii. Forced acid diuresis in poisoning with amphetamine, phencyclidine, quinine, etc. It can be done by administering mannitol or frusemide with ascorbic acid.
   b. Dialysis or hemoperfusion is helpful for extracorporeal removal of drugs and toxins.
   c. Exchange blood transfusion.
6. Care following withdrawal from alcohol or drugs:
7. Nursing care: Proper monitoring of vital signs, care of mouth and eyes, feeding, IV infusion, emptying of bladder, fluid, electrolyte balance, skin care, etc.

Barbiturate Poisoning

Short-acting barbiturates are more toxic than long-acting drugs. Long-acting drugs like phenobarbitone and barbitone are mostly excreted through kidneys. Ingestion of more than 6 gm of such drugs may be fatal. Short-acting drugs like phentobarbitone and secobarbitone are mostly metabolized in liver and ingestion of 3 gm of these drugs may be fatal.

Clinical Manifestations

1. Central nervous system depresssion. Altered consciousness.
2. Cardiovascular depression. Circulatory failure.
3. Respiratory depression.
4. Coma.
5. Confirmation of diagnosis by estimation of serum barbiturate levels. A level of 3.5 mg/100 ml with a long-acting drug or 8 mg/100 ml with the others indicates severe poisoning.

Management

1. No specific antidote.
2. General supportive measures.
3. Gastric lavage.
4. Respiratory care: Care of the airway, IPPV. Adequate oxygenation.
5. Cardiovascular support: IV infusions and vasopressors.
6. Antibiotics.
7. Forced alkaline diuresis.
8. Dialysis: Peritoneal or hemodialysis.
9. Tubefeeding, fluid, and electrolyte balance.
10. Body temperature may either fall or rise. This should be treated accordingly.

Salicylate Poisoning

Aspirin poisoning is common and dangerous with a significant mortality. Acute ingestion of more than 150 mg/kg or 10 gm in an adult causes toxicity and 500 mg/kg is potentially lethal. Salicylic acid readily passes into central nervous system and other tissues and tissue distribution is enhanced by acidosis. It is metabolized in liver and the metabolites and free salicylate are excreted through kidneys.

4. Coagulation abnormalities, gastrointestinal bleeding, pulmonary edema, and renal failure.
5. Respiratory failure and cardiovascular collapse.
6. Diagnosis is confirmed by blood salicylate levels. A level of over 3.6 mmol/L in adults and 2.1 mmol/L indicates for active therapy. Levels over 8.6 mmol/L carry poor prognosis.

Management

1. Gastric lavage.
2. Correction of metabolic acidosis. Sodium bicarbonate IV is indicated.
3. Forced alkaline diuresis.
4. Hemodialysis and hemoperfusion.
5. Supportive measures to correct hypovolemia, hyperpyrexia, hypoglycemia, hypokalemia, and hypoprothrombinemia, if present.

Paracetamol Poisoning

Paracetamol is being widely used as analgesic for treatment of headache, dysmenorrhea and for pain relief. Poisoning can occur when used in large amounts. It causes acute hepatic failure and its mortality rate is significant.

Clinical Features

1. Nausea, vomiting and abdominal pain.
2. Jaundice may appear within 4–5 days.
3. Liver is enlarged and tender.
4. Liver failure.
5. Renal failure.
6. Biochemical findings:
    a. Paracetamol levels of blood.

b. Liver function tests: SGOT, SGPT level increases. Bilirubin content is high.

Management

1. Supportive therapy.
2. Prevention can be tried by giving acetylcysteine.

Paracetamol causes liver damage due to its potentially toxic metabolites. These metabolites are usually made harmless by conjugation with glutathione in liver cells. In overdose the glutathione is depleted and liver damage occurs. Acetylcysteine prevents glutathione depletion and also inhibits the production of toxic metabolites. However, the drug should be given within 15 hours of ingestion, otherwise the damaged liver will be unable to metabolize it and hepatic coma may occur.

Tricyclic Antidepressants Poisoning

Various tricyclic antedepressants such as amitryptyline, imipramine, nortryptiline, doxepin, etc. are being widely used and poisoning by these drugs can occur.

Common toxic effects include anticholinergic effect, sympathomimetic effect, direct quinidine like myocardial effect and peripheral IV adrenergic blocking effect.

These drugs are mostly metabolized in liver and their metabolites are excreted through kidneys. They also undergo enterohepatic recirculation. Lethal dose is generally greater than 35 mg/kg.

Clinical Manifestations

1. Altered mental status. Agitation, confusion, delirium, stupor, coma, and convulsion.
2. Respiratory depression and pulmonary edema.

3. Dry mucous membrane and urinary retention.
4. Cardiovascular effects: Supraventricular or ventricular arrhythmias, conduction defect, hypertension, and hypotension.

Management

1. Monitoring of vital signs at frequent intervals.
2. Intensive supportive care.
3. Activated charcoal may help in rapid removal of the drug.
4. Hypotension: IV infusion of fluid and noradrenaline IV.
5. Ventricular arrhythmia: Lignocaine and phenytoin.
6. Supraventricular tachyarrhythmias: Physostigmine.
7. Conduction block: Phenytoin may help.
8. Convulsion: Diazepam, barbiturates may be needed to control it.

Lithium Poisoning

Lithium salts are being used in the management of manic-depressive psychosis. The margin between therapeutic and toxic levels is usually narrow. Severe toxic effects may be seen, if levels are above 3 mmol/L.

Clinical Features

1. Diarrhea, vomiting, thirst, polyuria, and tremor.
2. Vertigo, dysarthria, ataxia, and convulsion.
3. Coma.

Management

1. General supportive care.
2. Osmotic diuresis.
3. Alkalinization of urine.

4. Peritoneal or hemodialysis.
 5. Lithium level should be monitored for several days as diffusion from body tissues may cause rebound rise of lithium level.

Narcotic Poisoning

Common drugs used in narcotic poisoning are opium, morphine, pethidine, codeine, pentazocine, dextropropoxyphene, etc.

Chief Manifestations

1. Gross respiratory and cardiovascular depression.
2. Deep coma.
3. Pinpointed pupil.
4. Hypotension and bradycardia.
5. Presence of morphine or some other narcotic in urine confirms the diagnosis.
6. Barbiturates and alcohol worsen narcotic poisoning.

Management

1. Intense supportive care.
2. Gastric lavage and irrigation when taken orally.
3. Artificial ventilation and adequate oxygenation.
4. IV infusion of fluid.
5. Care of the unconscious patient.
6. Administration of antidote:
   a. Nalorphine 3–5 mg IV in small incremental doses.
   b. Levallorphan 1–3 mg IV in small incremental doses.
   c. Naloxone is more potent. Dose is 0.4 mg IM or IV and it can be repeated to a total three doses within a few minutes.
7. General supportive measures. Nutritional care.
8. Complications like pulmonary edema, infection, etc. should be treated accordingly.

Poisoning with Various Tranquilizers

Various phenothiazines and benzodiazepines are widely prescribed for various reasons. Poisoning may occur due to accidental overdose or as a suicidal attempt.

Common phenothiazines used are chlorpromazine, promethazine, trifluopromazine, trifluoperazine, etc. Benzodiazepines commonly used include diazepam, oxazepam, chlordiazepoxide, lorazepam, nitrazepam, etc.

Clinical Features

1. Drowsiness, light coma, nystagmus, dysarthria, and hypotension.
2. Phenothiazine in particular may cause coma, hypotension, hypothermia, dyskinetic movements, torticolis, convulsion, etc. Agranulocytosis can also occur.

Management

1. Gastric lavage.
2. Adequate oxygenation, maintenance of clear airway, and IPPV.
3. Cardiovascular support: Vasopressors and IV fluids.
4. Moderate diuresis to ensure urinary excretion of the drug.
5. General supportive measures care of the unconscious patient. Nutritional care.
6. Extrapyramidal reactions: Diphenhydramine, benztropinemesylate.
7. Arrhythmias: Lignocaine and phenytoin.

Organophosphorus Poisoning

1. Organophosphorus compounds are widely used as insecticides in agriculture. Parathion and malathion are used as pesticides.

2. Accidental or even suicidal poisoning can occur.
3. These are permanent anticholinesterase drugs and thus can cause accumulation of acetylcholine in different parts of the body.

Clinical Manifestations

1. Both nicotinic and muscarinic effects.
2. Respiratory insufficiency, bronchospasm, and pulmonary edema.
3. Excessive secretion, salivation, nausea, vomiting, sweating, fasciculations, myosis, and abdominal pain.
4. Bradycardia and hypotension.
5. Headache, tremor, slurred speech, ataxia, restlessness, confusion, and delirium.
6. Hyperthermia and convulsion.
7. Respiratory failure, cardiovascular collapse, and coma.

Management

1. Self-protection against chemicals, removal of contaminated clothings, and washing of the affected skin.
2. Maintenance of clear airway, IPPV, and adequate oxygenation.
3. IV infusion of fluids.
4. Atropinization 2 mg IV every 10 minutes till early atropine toxicity (dilated pupil, tachycardia, and restlessness) appears; thereafter, in reduced doses for several days.
5. Pralidoxime (a specific reactivator to cholinesterase) 1–2 gm slowly IV in addition to atropine.
6. General supportive measure.
7. Anticonvulsive therapy: Diazepam may be indicated.

Alcohol Poisoning

Ethyl Alcohol

Large quantities of alcohol can cause poisoning. In suicidal cases it is usually taken with other agents particularly barbiturates. Severe accidental poisoning can occur in children and severe hypoglycemia can result. Blood levels over 350 mg% may indicate severe toxicosis.

Clinical Features

Vomiting, ataxia, nystagmus, slurred speech, shock, hypothermia, hypoglycemia, lactic acidosis, respiratory depression, and coma.

Management

1. Gastric lavage.
2. In cases of of hypoglycemia—IV glucose.
3. Hemodialysis in severe cases.
4. For uncomplicated intoxication, only observation is needed.

Methyl Alcohol

It is cheap and is often used as substitute for ethyl alcohol by alcoholics who cannot afford ethyl alcohol. It may also be taken by mistake.

Clinical Features

1. Severe acidosis due to its metabolite formic acid.
2. Rapid respiration, cyanosis, and hypotension.
3. Headache, vertigo, and coma.
4. Acute visual disturbances and optic neuritis.
5. Hypoglycemia.
6. Fatal dose may be 60–250 ml.

Management

1. Gastric lavage.
2. Acidosis: Sodium bicarbonate, etc.

3. Hemodialysis in severe cases when blood level is above 50 mg%.
4. General supportive measures.
5. Ethyl alcohol IV may give some protection against methyl alcohol poisoning by reducing its metabolism to formaldehyde and formic acid.

Carbon Monoxide Poisoning

Carbon monoxide is produced by the incomplete combustion of carbon or carbonaceous materials and is released by fires, faulty stoves or heating systems. Car exhausts are potent source of carbon monoxide. Fire in small rooms with inefficient ventilation is dangerous. This may occur in suicidal attempts or accidents in course of fires.

Hemoglobin has great affinity for carbon monoxide and the resulting carboxyhemoglobin is incapable to carry oxygen and severe tissue hypoxia occurs.

Clinical Manifestations

1. Hypoxemia (anemic hypoxia).
2. Headache, restlessness, dizziness, and weakness.
3. Nausea and vomiting.
4. Dyspnea.
5. Ataxia, cerebral edema, convulsion, and coma.
6. Confirmation of diagnosis by the assessment of blood carboxyhemoglobin concentration.
7. Complications of carbon monoxide poisoning may include psychological problems, neurological deficit, myocardial ischemia or infarction.

Management

1. Intensive supportive care, and removal from polluted atmosphere.

2. Ventilation with 100% oxygen and IPPV.
3. Sodium bicarbonate IV to combat metabolic acidosis.
4. Adequate artificial ventilation to treat respiratory acidosis.
5. General supportive measures.
6. Shock and cerebral edema should be treated accordingly.

Cyanide Poisoning

Cyanides are commonly used in industry. Hydrogen cyanide is used as a fumigant, cyanamide as fertilizer and other salts in metal cleaning and ore extraction processes. When a strong acid reacts with cyanide salts, hydrocyanic acid is liberated and it can cause poisoning.

Cyanide inhibits the cytochrome oxidase system for oxygen utilization and acts as cellular poison. Following ingestion or inhalation, coma, and death occurs within seconds from respiratory paralysis.

Management

1. Instant treatment is needed for survival of the patient.
2. IPPV and adequate oxygenation.
3. Cobalt tetracemate by rapid IV injection.
4. Sodium nitrite IV followed by sodium thiosulfate IV may also help.
5. General supportive care.

Poisoning with Amphetamines

These are potent central nervous system and sympathetic stimulants. Ingestion of 20–25 mg/kg may cause death.

Clinical Manifestations

1. Hyperactivity, irritability, and delirium.

2. Hypertension and cardiac arrhythmias.
3. Vomiting and diarrhea.
4. Mydriasis.
5. Hyperpyrexia.
6. Cerebrovascular hemorrhage, convulsion, and coma.
7. Shock and cardiovascular collapse.
8. Acute renal failure.
9. Coagulation disorders.

Management

1. Gastric lavage, activated charcoal, and cathartic.
2. Forced acid diuresis.
3. Hemodialysis in severe cases.
4. Intensive supportive care.
5. Treatment of complications:
   a. Agitation and pyschosis—Haloperidol and diazepam.
   b. Arrhythmias—Propranolol.
   c. Hypertension—Chlorpromazine, diazoxide, phentolamine, and sodium nitroprusside.

Cocaine Poisoning

It is a potent and powerful central nervous system and sympathetic stimulant. It is usually taken by nasal insufflation. It can also be used by smoking or IV injection. But it is not taken orally as oral absorption is poor due to gastric hydrolysis.

Clinical Features

1. Excitability, restlessness, mydriasis, tachycardia, hypertension, and cardiac arrhythmias.
2. Hyperthermia.
3. Convulsion.
4. Respiratory failure.

5. Shock and cardiovascular failure.
6. Coma.
7. Diagnosis may be confirmed by blood and urine level estimations.

Management

1. Intensive supportive care.
2. Care of the airway, adequate oxygenation, and IPPV.
3. IV infusion of fluids.
4. Diazepam to treat and control convulsion.
5. Propranolol to treat adrenergic phenomena.

Poisoning by Toxic Irritant Gases

There may be accidental exposure of various noxious gases such as chlorine, ammonia, formaldehyde, sulfur dioxide, phosgene, nitrogen dioxide and so on. These may cause local irritation, asphyxiation and systemic toxicity. Depending upon the degree and duration of exposure, these may cause significant morbidity and mortality.

Clinical Features

1. Cutaneous burns, irritation to the mucosa, laryngotracheitis, bronchitis, bronchospasm, pulmonary edema, and upper airway obstruction.
2. Shock and cardiovascular failure.
3. Respiratory failure.

Management

1. Removal of the victim in a safe atmosphere.
2. Establishment of a patent airway, IPPV, and adequate oxygenation.
3. Humidified oxygen may be helpful.

4. Noncardiogenic pulmonary edema—Oxygen, IPPV with the use of positive end-expiratory pressure.
5. Bronchospasm: Bronchodilators.
6. Care of the eyes.
7. Some investigations like arterial blood gas analysis, chest radiograph, etc. may be beneficial.
8. Shock: IV infusion, vasopressors, and steroids.
9. Skin burns: Local cleansing, aseptic dressing, and tetanus prophylaxis.
10. The offending agent should be identified and measures should be taken accordingly.

Poisoning with Caustics

These are mostly accidental but may be suicidal. Both acids and alkalis cause serious problems by producing burns and necrosis with significant morbidity and mortality.

Clinical Features

1. Pain in mouth, oropharynx, chest, and abdomen
2. Dysphagia
3. Respiratory distress and upper airway edema
4. Aspiration pneumonitis
5. Gastrointestinal bleeding and perforation may also occur
6. Mediastinitis and peritonitis
7. Airway obstruction
8. Shock and circulatory collapse.

Management

1. Dilution: Mouth should be washed with a large volume of cold water. In cases of alkali, milk or water may be allowed to swallow. In acid ingestion this swallowing is not advised as it might cause exothermic reaction.

2. Induced emesis and gastric lavage are contraindicated in caustic ingestion.
3. Activated charcoal and cathartic are also not recommended.
4. Establishment of clear airway. Adequate oxygenation and IPPV.
5. Adequate fluid management.
6. Monitoring of vital signs: Examination for any gastrointestinal hemorrhage and/or perforation. Careful endoscopy may be helpful.
7. Nutritional care.
8. General supportive cares.

# Chapter 9

Cardiopulmonary Resuscitation

Cardiopulmonary Arrest

Cardiopulmonary arrest implies the cessation of spontaneous and effective cardiac output and ventilation. Cardiopulmonary resuscitation is a series of well-defined guidelines and protocol for management of such cases to provide artificial circulation and ventilation.

- It is indicated most commonly for severely low cardiac output states, cardiac arrest, respiratory arrest or a combination of both.

Cardiopulmonary arrest may have some probable causative factors:

1. Anesthesia: Overdose of anesthetic and analgesic drugs, bad anesthesia associated with hypoxia, hypercarbia and hypotension. Use of cardiotoxic anesthetic drugs.
2. Severe hypoxia, hypercarbia, and hypotension from any cause. Major trauma, acute hypovolemia, and shock.
3. Toxicity of local anesthetic drugs, digitalis, quinidine, and procainamide.
4. Severe electrolyte changes.
5. Severe acid-base disturbances.

6. Some cardiac diseases: Heart block, valvular diseases, coronary occlusion, myocardial infarction, myocarditis, cardiomyopathy, cardiac failure, and cardiac tamponade.
7. Instrumentations: Cardiac catheterization, and bronchoscopy.
8. Embolisms.
9. Hyperthermia and hypothermia.
10. Anaphylaxis.
11. Uremia and toxemia.
12. Electric shock, electrocution, direct myocardial contact with the electrocautery.
13. Drowning.
14. Acute spinal injury.
15. Head injury, chest injury, and abdominal injury.
16. Poisoning.

Diagnosis of Cardiopulmonary Arrest

1. Sudden disappearance of pulse even in great vessels, like femoral and carotid arteries.
2. Absence of heart beat/precordial heart sounds.
3. No respiration and gasping.
4. Unconsciousness.
5. Widely dilated pupils and unresponsive to light.
6. Electrocardiogram:
   a. Asystole, no contraction of myocardium.
   b. Ventricular fibrillation: Uncoordinated and ineffectual contraction of myocardium.
   c. There may be QRS complex on ECG, but no palpable pulse (electromechanical dissociation).

Management

Brain tolerates only 3–4 minutes of anoxia before succumbing to permanent damage. So early diagnosis and vigorous treatment are mandatory and no time should be wasted. But in hyperthermic, toxic, and hypoxic patients permanent brain damage may occur even in a much shorter period. The most common cause of death in such cases is undue delay in starting resuscitation; so when circulatory arrest has occurred, cardiopulmonary resuscitation (CPR) should be commenced instantly.

Management of CPR needs consideration in two stages:
1. Rapid initiation and continuation of basic life support to provide artificial circulation and ventilation by simple maneuvers.
2. Advanced cardiac life support with the use of advanced techniques of mechanical ventilation and artificial circulation.

Basic Life Support

1. Call for help and utilize all helps available. Initiate immediate life support measures. Utilize professional knowledge skillfully.
2. **Provision of a patent airway**: Head-tilt chin-lift maneuver helps to relieve obstruction due to the tongue falling against posterior pharynx. The jaw thrust maneuver without head-tilt is useful for opening the airway in a subject with a suspected neck (cervical) injury.
3. **Expired air ventilation**: Ventilation should be commenced either mouth-to-mouth or mouth-to-nose breathing. The patient's mouth is covered by the mouth of the rescuer while the patient's nostrils are pinched, closed and the rescuer blows his expired air into the patient, until his chest starts to rise. Then the rescuer stops blowing, removes his mouth and allows the patient to exhale. Ventilation rate should be 12–15 times per minute. One inflation every 5 cycles of cardiac compression is required.

Expired air ventilation can also be done by mouth-to-nose where mouth is kept closed and ventilation is carried through nose of the patient and then the patient's mouth is opened to permit passive expiration to occur. In neonates and infants, both the mouth and nose can be used at a time for such ventilation.
- Problems of such expired air ventilation include esthetic side of the technique, failure to maintain a patent airway, failure to keep an airtight seal, gastric distension, and regurgitation.

4. **External cardiac massage**: The patient is placed supine on firm surface. Cardiac massage is to be given by placing one hand over the lower-half or third of the sternum and the second hand over the first one. Then the rescuer leans forward to transmit his weight of the upper body to patient's thorax. Arms should be kept straight to reduce fatigue. The sternum is depressed 1.5–2 inches (4–5 cm) along with the heart against vertebra. This is repeated 80 times per minute. Equal time should be allowed for each compression and relaxation. Effective massage will carry the impulse to the big vessels.

   a. In case of children, it is recommended to use one hand on a midsternal position and the compression rate is 100–120 times per minute. In neonates, the force by only two fingers is enough. In the baby the compression ventilation ratio is kept to 5 : 1 and the compression depth is 1.5 cm and the compression rate is 100/min.

   b. External chest compression may result in 60–100 mmHg and a cardiac output of 20%–50% of normal. But complications like fracture of ribs, sternum or vertebra, rupture of spleen or liver, and injury of heart or pericardium may occur. It is contraindicated

in presence of cardiac tamponade, tension pneumothorax or uncontrolled intrathoracic hemorrhage.
c. To maintain effective ventilation during closed chest cardiac massage, it is essential to coordinate two maneuvers. When 2 operators are available, one should give 4 cardiac compressions and allow the other for 1 mouth-to-mouth breathing. For one single operator, 2 successive inflations should be followed by 8 successive cardiac compressions.
d. In new technique the two maneuvers are timed to coincide. This may cause cyclical increase in intrathoracic pressure and thereby may increase the forward flow of blood. Here, the cardiac compressions should be performed continuously and not interrupted during lung inflations. Repeatedly assess and re-evaluate the condition of the patient.

Advanced Cardiac Life Support

It includes the use of various equipment and techniques of ventilation and cardiac resuscitation.

1. **Airway**:
   a. Clear the mouth and upper airway by suction.
   b. Oropharyngeal or nasopharyngeal airway.
   c. Endotracheal intubation.
2. **Ventilation**:
   a. Use of self-inflating resuscitation bag (Ambu bag) with oxygen-enriched air.
   b. IPPV with 100% oxygen.
   c. Mechanical ventilators for prolonged ventilation.
3. **Circulation**:
   a. Mechanical chest thumpers may be helpful to restart cardiac rhythm.

b. Pharmacological.
c. Internal cardiac massage. Transabdominal or transthoracic route.

A large incision in the left fourth or fifth intercostal space is made starting 1 inch away from sternum to avoid the injury to internal mammary artery upto midaxillary line. Lungs are retracted and the heart along with pericardium should be lifted. Then the heart should be compressed between both palms 50–60 times per minute. Heart should be watched for diagnosis either of asystole or ventricular fibrillation. The technique needs skilled personnel and special instruments. It needs positive pressure ventilation.

Internal cardiac massage is very effective and the heart can be directly seen and the type of arrest can be judged. Intracardiac injection of adrenaline can be better given. Internal defibrillation can also be better performed. In cases of cardiac tamponade, internal massage is possible after relieving the tamponade.

Pharmacological Support

Electrocardiogram should be done to diagnose the type of cardiac arrest: ventricular fibrillation, cardiac asystole or electromechanical dissociation.

Ventricular Fibrillation

1. Immediate DC countershock of 200 joules.
2. Repeat second time with 200 joules.
3. Then a third time with 360 joules if ventricular fibrillation persists.
4. If unsuccessful give adrenaline (1 ml of a 1 : 1000 solution or 10 ml of a 1 : 10000 solution) IV and then defibrillation with 360 joules using different paddle positions.

5. Other antiarrhythmic drug (lignocaine 100 ml) may be used.
6. Use of sodium bicarbonate may be considered to combat acidosis.

Cardiac Asystole

1. Give adrenaline 1 mg IV.
2. Atropine sulfate 2 mg IV.
3. Internal pacing.
4. If ventricular fibrillation cannot be excluded, it is better to defibrillate first with 200 joules, repeat with 200 joules and then with 360 joules and then gives adrenaline and consider pacing.

Electromechanical Dissociation

Causes

1. *Primary causes*:
   a. Severe myocardial infarction
   b. Overdose of β-blockers and calcium antagonists
   c. Toxins
   d. Hypocalcemia
   e. Hyperkalemia.
2. *Secondary causes*:
   a. Massive trauma
   b. Hypovolemia
   c. Massive pulmonary embolism
   d. Tension pneumothorax
   e. Pericardial tamponade
   f. Prosthetic heart valve malfunction.

Management

QRS complex present, but without palpable pulse.
1. Give adrenaline 1 mg IV.

2. Specific therapy for hypovolemia, pneumothorax, pulmonary embolism, etc.
3. Calcium chloride 10 ml 10% to treat hyperkalemia, hypocalcemia and overdose of calcium antagonists.

Additional Measures to be Taken

1. IV fluid—Fluid replacement.
2. Correction of metabolic acidosis. Sodium bicarbonate.
3. Vasopressors.
4. Dopamine.
5. Oxygen therapy.
6. Digitalization, β-blockers, etc.
7. Sodium bicarbonate—Dose should be titrated with blood gas analysis.

Special Note

1. Bicarbonate is indicated:
   a. Measured pH less than 7.2.
   b. Pre-existing metabolic acidosis.
   c. Tricyclic antedepressant/barbiturate overdose.
   d. Empirically when blood gas analysis unobtainable.
2. Calcium therapy:
   a. Intracellular Ca excess may cause cellular injury and death.
   b. Indicated in hyperkalemia/hypocalcemia overdose of Ca-channel blockers.
   c. Dose: 2–4 mg/kg of calcium chloride may be repeated every 10 minutes.

Post-treatment Complications

Follow-up care after the crisis:
1. Cerebral edema—Brain damage.
2. Pulmonary edema.

3. Kidney failure.
4. Cardiovascular problems:
   a. Myocardial infarction
   b. Pulmonary embolism
   c. Hypovolemia
   d. Arrhythmias.
5. Neurological problems:
   a. Success of CPR depends on:
      i. Pre-existing condition of the patient
      ii. Immediate diagnosis
      iii. Instant basic cardiac life support
      iv. Advanced cardiac life support
      v. Dedicated expert team work.
   b. Termination of CPR may be considered: (if law permits)
      i. Permanent brain damage and brain death.
      ii. Terminal stages of incurable diseases.
      iii. Gross congenital defects.
      iv. Likelihood of seminormality.
      v. Second expert opinion is mandatory.
      vi. Document the event in record.
   c. Criteria for brain death in an adult in the absence of hypothermia (below 32°C) or overdose of depressant drugs or both are:
      i. Coma persisting more than 12 hours in presence of a known disease.
      ii. Absent brainstem function:
         – Fixed and unreactive pupils.
         – Apnea despite increase $PaCO_2$.
         – Absent vestibulo-ocular reflex.
         – No motor response within cranial nerve distribution.
         – No corneal reflex/gag reflex.
      iii. Absent cortical function (flat EEG).
      iv. Absent cerebral circulation in angiography.

Chapter 10

Fluid, Electrolyte and Acid-base Disorders

Disturbancess of fluid, electrolyte, and acid-base balance are common in patients of critical care unit. Hemorrhages, shock, sepsis, gastrointestinal fluid losses, hyperpyrexia, hypothermia diabetes, diuresis, trauma, central nervous system injury, burns, hypoxia, respiratory failure, liver failure, renal failure, etc. can cause such disorders. Thorough clinical examination, urine and blood examination, blood biochemistry, serum electrolytes estimation arterial blood gas analysis, etc. should be monitored for early detection and management.

Dehydration

Simple and uncomplicated dehydration is a reduction of total water content of the body due to loss of sodium and water.

Causes

1. From gastrointestinal tract: Severe diarrhea, excessive vomiting, cholera, ulcerative colitis, etc.
2. Excessive sweating
3. Urinary loss: Addison's disease, diabetes mellitus, salt losing nephritis, excessive diuretics, etc.

4. Hyperpyrexia
5. Severe hemorrhage
6. Hyperventilation: Increased loss of water from lung.

Manifestations

Thirst, oliguria, decreased skin turgor. Sunken eyeball, dry mucous membrane, low central venous pressure, hypotension, and tachycardia.

Impaired kidney function; BUN: Creatinine ratio more than 20, urinary specific gravity and osmolality increased, urinary sodium decreased. Volume deficit may be mild, moderate and severe when there is loss of 4%, 6%, and 8% of body weight respectively.

Plasma shows low volume, raised protein levels, increased PCV, high Hb concentration, high blood viscosity, increased specific gravity, low plasma sodium, and high blood urea.

Management

1. Indentify the cause of volume loss, if possible and treat accordingly.
2. Volume replacement with normal saline, blood or colloid as indicated.
3. Blood transfusion in cases of massive blood loss.
4. Gencral supportive care.

Pure Water-deficiency

It is rare but can occur in direct deprivation of water as in esophageal obstruction, starvation, shipwreck, etc. loss of water in diabetes insipidus or when water is unavailable.

Manifestations

1. Thirst, rise of body temperature, and mental impairment.

2. Urine: Low volume and high specific gravity.
3. Plasma: Increased sodium and potassium. Hb concentration and PCV mostly unchanged due to loss of water from RBC.
4. Ultimately hypotension and coma occur due to intracellular dehydration to vital organs.

Management

1. Nonsaline fluids IV or orally
2. General supportive care.

Water Intoxication (Excess)

It can occur when there is an increase in total body water without comparable increase of total body sodium.

Cause

1. Over infusion.
2. Anuria/oliguria: Intake is normal but little or no urinary output.
3. Large intake of fluid but kidneys fail to compensate with diuresis: Excessive ADH, severe liver disease, head injury, etc.

Effect

Initially it will lead to diuresis, but later the renal cells are damaged resulting oliguria and anuria. Extracellular compartment is distended and its osmolarity is reduced. Excess water goes into cells to cause intracellular edema, ultimately there will be edema in lungs, skin, brain, muscles, and widespread cellular damage all over the body.

Manifestation

1. Initially increase in body weight, increased central venous pressure, high pulse pressure, swollen eyelids,

exertional dyspnea, engorged neck, veins, diuresis, cyanosis, coughing, etc.
2. Acute intoxication: Nausea/vomiting, weakness, muscle cramps, headache, dizziness, apathy, stupor, convulsion, and coma.
3. Chronic intoxication: Pulmonary edema and systemic edema.

Management

1. Treat the underlying cause.
2. Restriction of fluid and electrolytes.
3. Judicious administration of diuretics.
4. Hypertonic 5% saline or molar 5.85% saline given IV slowly.
5. Strict monitoring of vital signs.
6. General supportive care.

Hypercalcemia

Hypercalcemia (plasma calcium levels in excess of 5.5 mEq/L) may require urgent treatment as it may provoke a dangerous hypercalcemic crisis which carries a high mortality rate.

Causes

1. Malignancy (metastatic carcinoma).
2. Primary hyperparathyroidism.
3. Sarcoidosis.
4. Vitamin D intoxication.
5. Milk alkalis syndrome.
6. Adrenal insufficiency.
7. Hyperthyroidism.
8. Prolonged immobilization.
9. Hypophosphatemia.

Clinical Manifestations

1. Central nervous system: Headache, lethargy, psychosis, muscle weakness, confusion, and coma.
2. Renal: Thirst, polyuria, renal calculus, dehydration, and renal dysfunction.
3. Gastrointestinal: Nausea, vomiting, abdominal pain, constipation, peptic ulcer, and acute pancreatitis.
4. Cardiovascular: Hypertension, various ECG changes, cardiac conduction disturbances (prolonged P-R interval, wide QRS, shortened QT interval).
5. Clinical features of primary disease: Bone pain, etc.

Diagnosis

1. Serum calcium estimation.
2. ECG.

Management

It mainly depends on the underlying cause and the degrees of renal dysfunction. In primary hyperparathyroidism, parathyroidectomy is indicated. In malignant bone disease, radiotherapy or cytotoxic agents are indicated, but emergency treatment is required to save the patient.

Treatment

1. Rehydration.
2. Diuresis: Normal saline plus furosemide, in presence of CVP monitoring. Adequate water and electrolyte replacement is essential. Overzealous use of furosemide is harmful.
3. Glucocorticoids may be helpful in cases with lymphoma, multiple myeloma, vitamin D intoxication, etc.

4. Calcitonin: It is the treatment of choice in presence of renal dysfunction. It lowers serum calcium by inhibiting resorption of bone calcium. It also inhibits renal tubular reabsorption.
5. Sodium phosphate supplementation may be helpful. But metastatic calcification can occur and it may be dangerous in cases with renal impairment.
6. Mithramycin: This cytotoxic agent has been used for the emergency treatment. But it has marked bone marrow toxic effects.
7. Peritoneal dialysis/hemodialysis.

Hypocalcemia

Hypocalcemia may also cause serious problems and often requires early treatment. Hypocalcemia occurs when plasma calcium concentration is below 4.5 mEq/L.

Causes

1. Decreased plasma albumin concentration.
2. Hypoparathyroidism and removal of parathyroids.
3. Renal failure.

Clinical Manifestations

1. Muscle cramps and paresthesia in extremities and around the mouth.
2. Severe spasms, bronchospasm, carpopedal spasm, and tetany.
3. Cramps in jaws, respiratory muscles and laryngeal muscles often lead to acute respiratory insufficiency.
4. Dementia, toxic delirium, convulsion, restlessness, and coma.
5. Papilledema and hypotension.
6. Plasma calcium estimation confirms the diagnosis. Serum calcium less than 8 mg/100 ml.

7. ECG changes: Prolonged Q-T interval. Atrial and ventricular arrhythmias.

Treatment

1. Treat the underlying cause.
2. Intravenous infusion of calcium. Calcium gluconate 10%.
3. Correction of any coexisting alkalosis.
4. Note: Hypokalemia and hypomagnesemia potentiate the cardiac and neuromuscular effects of hypocalcemia. Magnesium sulfate may often be needed.
5. For chronic management, oral calcium supplementation and vitamin D supplementation are advised.
6. Frequent monitoring of serum calcium is essential.

Hyperkalemia

Hyperkalemia is a serious problem and it needs early detection and treatment. Hyperkalemia occurs when serum potassium concentration is more than 5.5 mEq/L.

Causes

1. Due to increased total body potassium content:
   a. Acute oliguric renal failure.
   b. Chronic renal failure (later stage).
   c. Hypoaldosteronism—Adrenal insufficiency.
   d. Some drugs may impair potassium excretion: Triamterene, spironolactone, etc.
   e. Some drugs inhibit the renin-angiotensin aldosterone system: β-antagonists, and ACE inhibitors.
   f. Crush injury, massive trauma, and burns.
2. Due to alteration in distribution of potassium between intracellular and extracellular fluid compartments:
   a. Suxamethonism.

b. Respiratory or metabolic acidosis.
c. Hemolysis, massive blood transfusion, lysis of red blood cells.
d. Malignant hyperthermia.
e. Hyperkalemic periodic paralysis.
f. Massive administration of potassium.
3. Pseudohyperkalemia is due to the in vitro release of intracellular potassium.

Clinical Manifestations and Diagnosis

1. Acute increase in serum potassium concentration. Serum potassium above 5.5 mEq/L.
2. ECG changes: Cardiac conduction disturbances, complete heart block, prolongation of PR interval, widening of the QRS complex, tall peaked T-waves with narrow base. Ventricular fibrillation may occur. It should be noted that ECG changes do not appear until serum potassium rises above 6.5 mEq/L.

Treatment

1. Avoid potassium administration. Confirm diagnosis. Check ECG.
2. Correction of hypoxia and adequate oxygenation.
3. Hyperventilation—$PaCO_2$ should be between 25 and 30 mmHg.
4. Use of ion exchange resins by rectal or oral routes in cases of mild hyperkalemia.
5. Sodium bicarbonate 50–150 mEq IV treat underlying metabolic acidosis, if present.
6. Calcium gluconate 10–20 ml of a 10% solution IV.
7. Glucose and insulin infusion 20–50 gm glucose with 10–20 units of insulin IV.
8. Forced diuresis—Frusemide.

9. Peritoneal dialysis.
10. Hemodialysis: Avoid rapid correction. Monitor serum potassium, urine output, and cardiac rhythms.

Chronic Hyperkalemia may be Treated

1. Dietary restriction of potassium
2. Diuretic therapy: Loop diuretics and thiazides
3. Oral bicarbonate replacement
4. Fludrocortisone acetate
5. Cation exchange resins.

Complications

1. Arrhythmias.
2. Ventricular fibrillation.
3. Hyperosmolality, hypoglycemia, hypokalemia may also occur as complications of therapy. Dialysis-related problems may also occur.

Hypokalemia

Hypokalemia occurs when plasma potassium concentration is below 3.5 mEq/L. Acute hypokalemia is a serious problem for patient's safety while chronic cases are less significant.

Causes

1. Decreased total body potassium content:
a. Gastrointestinal loss: Diarrhea, laxative abuse, intestinal or biliary fistula, vomiting, and nasogastric suction.
b. Urinary loss: Diuretics, some antibiotics like amphotericin, aminoglycosides, etc. renal tubular acidosis, hyperaldosteronism, glucocorticoid excess, magnesium deficiency, and surgical trauma.
c. Inadequate intake of potassium.

2. Altered distribution of potassium between intracellular and extracellular compartments.
   a. Respiratory or metabolic alkalosis.
   b. Glucose and insulin.
   c. Hypercalcemia.

Clinical Manifestations

1. *Neuromuscular disturbances*: Muscular cramps, weakness of muscles, hyporeflexia, paresthesia, and paralysis. Respiratory failure.
2. *Cardiovascular disturbances*: Arrhythmias, orthostatic hypotension, ECG changes—T-wave and U-waves flattening, ST segment depression. Cardiac conduction disturbances. Cardiac arrest.
3. *Uropathy*: Polyuria, polydipsia, and glucose intolerance.
4. *Others*: Constipation, paralytic ileus, metabolic alkalosis, and hyperglycemia.

Diagnosis

1. Serum potassium estimation. Serum potassium less than 3.5 mEq/L.
2. Electrocardiogram.

Management

1. It will depend on the etiology and degree of hypokalemia. Potassium supplementation should be guided by plasma potassium estimation periodically. Prevention of significant hypokalemia should be tried in patients with cardiac disease and those on digitalis therapy. Replacement of potassium is needed in patients receiving potassium wasting diuretics.
2. Excessive hyperventilation should be corrected.

Avoid conditions that reduce serum potassium acutely such as hyperventilation, metabolic alkalosis, β_2-adrenergic stimulation.
3. Supplemental potassium chloride is helpful in severely depleted patients.
   a. Oral potassium therapy: Potassium chloride may be given when oral absorption is normal.
   b. Potassium-rich foods, fruits, and vegetables.
   c. IV therapy: It may be added to intravenous infusions or continuous infusion as a therapeutic measure. Continuous ECG monitoring and measurement of serum potassium concentration every 4–6 hours should be performed. Urine output should also be monitored. IV therapy may be dangerous, if given too rapidly or in presence of renal impairment.
4. Treat underlying cause such as vomiting, alkalosis, etc.
5. Avoid elective surgery/anesthesia in presence of hypokalemia. Difficulty in reversing nondepolarizing muscle relaxants.

Complications

1. Hyperkalemia, cardiac arrhythmias or even cardiac arrest can occur due to excessive potassium replacement.
2. Respiratory failure and cardiac arrest.

Hypernatremia

Here the plasma sodium concentration exceeds more than 145 mEq/L. It is mostly due to a deficit of total body water and not to an excess of total body sodium. Kidneys closely regulate total body sodium content and excess sodium retention is not usually possible, unless there is impaired renal function as in cases with congestive heart failure, cirrhosis of liver, kidney failure, etc.

Causes

1. Hypotonic fluid loss and ECF volume contraction:
   a. Inadequate fluid intake
   b. Diarrhea
   c. Chronic renal failure
   d. Diabetes insipidus
   e. Diaphoresis
   f. Osmotic diuresis.
2. Hypertonic ECF volume expansion:
   a. Hypertonic sodium bicarbonate therapy
   b. High sodium intake without water supplement
   c. Hyperaldosteronism
   d. Cushing's syndrome
   e. Excessive steroid therapy for prolonged period.

Clinical Manifestations

These will mostly depend on the underlying cause and ECF volume status.

1. In cases with ECF volume contraction:
   a. State of dehydration.
   b. Mental confusion, irritability, tremor, convulsion, and coma.
2. In cases with ECF volume expansion:
   a. Peripheral edema and weight gain.
   b. Hypertension and tachycardia.
   c. Changes of mental status, changes of level of consciousness.
   d. Increased CVP and pulmonary pressures.
   e. Dyspnea, cough, and moist breath sounds.
   f. Urine output less.

Laboratory Findings

In cases with ECF volume contraction:
1. Increased hemoglobin content and hematocrit value.
2. Serum osmolality more than 295 mOsm/kg.
3. Serum sodium more than 145 mEq/L.
4. Urinary sodium less than 20 mEq/L.
5. Urine osmolality more than 500 mEq/L.
6. Specific gravity of urine more than 1015.

Management

1. Water deficit should be replaced.
2. Serum sodium estimation should be repeatedly evaluated. Plasma osmolality should be corrected slowly. Rapid correction may be detrimental.
3. In cases of ECF volume excess—
   a. Diuresis
   b. Dialysis in cases of renal failure
   c. Hypotonic IV fluids
   d. Sodium and fluid restriction.
4. In cases of ECF volume depletion—
   a. Sodium and fluid restriction.
   b. Fluid replacement therapy. Isotonic or hypotonic saline may be considered.
   c. Electrolyte replacement therapy.

Hyponatremia

Hyponatremia occurs when serum sodium concentration is below 124 mEq/L and/or abnormally low serum osmolality, less than 270 mOsm/L. It is a serious condition and needs early detection and treatment. It may be due to altered relationship of total body water to sodium or altered body water distribution due to osmotic effects.

Pseudohyponatremia with low serum sodium with normal or elevated osmolality can also occur.

Causes

1. Dilution of sodium:
   a. Cardiac failure.
   b. Nephrotic syndrome—Chronic renal failure.
   c. Hepatic insufficiency.
   d. Excessive hypotonic electrolyte-free IV infusion. Hemodilution. Following cystoscopic surgery.
   e. Syndrome of inappropriate ADH secretion.
2. Sodium loss:
   a. Diarrhea.
   b. Vomiting and nasogastric suctioning.
   c. Diuretic drugs—Thiazide diuretics.
   d. Adrenal insufficiency.
   e. Renal disease.
3. Pseudohyponatremia may occur in metabolic disorders as in hyperglycemia, hyperproteinemia, hyperlipidemia, etc.

Clinical Manifestations

The severity of clinical features depends on the degree of hyponatremia and rate of decrease of serum sodium concentration.

1. When there is sodium dilution—
   a. Headache, irritability, weakness, muscle cramps, and muscle twitching.
   b. Altered mental status and level of consciousness. Visual disturbances—Dyspnea.
   c. Convulsion.
   d. Cardiac, hepatic or renal dysfunction.
   e. Pulmonary or laryngeal edema. Intravascular hemolysis.

2. When there is sodium loss—
   a. Lethargy, confusion, headache, drowsy, and coma.
   b. Muscle cramps and convulsion.
   c. Postural hypotension and peripheral circulatory failure.

Laboratory Findings

1. Serum osmolality less than 270 mOsm/kg
2. Serum sodium less than 124 mEq/L
3. Urinary sodium more than 20 mEq/L.

Management

1. Hyponatremia with a decreased plasma osmolality:
   a. Hypovolemia with excess ECF volume and edema. Diuretics with sensible precautions. Hypertonic saline is not indicated in such cases and actually it may be hazardous.
   b. Hyponatremia with clinically normal ECF volume:
      i. Syndrome of inappropriate ADH secretion. In acute cases, rapid diuresis with IV frusemide followed by replacement of sodium and potassium lost in urine. Thereafter, water restriction is indicated. Demeclocycline therapy may be helpful. Frusemide and oral urea may also be effective.
      ii. Water intoxication—Rapid diuresis with IV frusemide. Replacement of sodium and potassium.
      iii. Hyponatremia with decreased ECF volume (vomiting, diarrhea, salt losing nephropathy, diuretic phase of acute tubular necrosis, osmotic diuresis, etc.) Re-expansion of ECF volume with isotonic saline. Correction of the underlying pathology.
2. Hyponatremia with a normal plasma osmolality or pseudohyponatremia (severe hyperlipidemia and

hyperproteinemia). No specific fluid and electrolyte therapy is needed.
3. Hyponatremia with an increase in osmotically active solutes (hyperglycemia).
   Reduction of ECF hypertonicity by correction of the underlying cause.

Prevention of Hyponatremia

1. Fluid replacement with hypotonic solutions should be avoided.
2. Electrolyte levels should be checked frequently in cases with renal failure, metabolic abnormalities and those undergoing major surgery.
3. Patients receiving drugs that can cause hyponatremia needs careful electrolyte estimations frequently.
4. Patients during transurethral resection of prostrate (TURP) need special attention:
   a. Sterile water as irrigation fluid should not be used.
   b. Resection time should be minimized.
   c. High irrigation pressure should be avoided.

Complications

1. Cerebral edema.
2. Hyperosmolality due to hypertonic saline therapy.
3. Central pontine myelinolysis or diffuse cerebral demyelination secondary to too rapid restoration of serum sodium.

Hyperphosphatemia

About 85% of total body phosphorus remains in bone and the rest is mostly within the cells as the major intracellular anion. Only 1% of the total body phosphorus is in the extracellular fluid, the serum phosphorus concentration cannot reflect total body phosphorus. Phosphorus is important in bone formation. It is an essential factor of adenosine triphosphate and thus essential for normal cellular metabolism. Its presence in red blood cell helps the hemoglobin oxygen affinity and tissue oxygen delivery. Phosphorus balance is maintained by parathyroid hormone, active vitamin D, and insulin.

Hyperphosphatemia is usually the result of impaired urinary excretion of PO_4 in patients with renal insufficiency. Increased PO_4 release from cells in cases of prominent cell necrosis as in tumorlysis, etc. Here serum phosphate level is above 5 mg/dL.

Clinical manifestations

1. Formation of insoluble calcium—Phosphate complexes with deposition in soft tissues, vasculature, cornea, kidney, and joints.
2. Acute hypocalcemia—Tetany may occur.

Management

1. Treat the underlying cause, whenever possible.
2. Aluminum-containing antacid may be used to bind phosphate in gastrointestinal system.
3. Forced saline resuscitation with addition of acetazolamide.
4. Dietary restriction.
5. Hemodialysis in refractory cases.

Hypophosphatemia

Here serum phosphate level is below 2.5 mg/dL. It is severe if the level is below 1 mg/dL. To evaluate a case with hypophosphatemia, severe vitamin D-deficiency and primary hyperparathyroidism should be excluded. The other causes are as follow:

1. Gastrointestinal losses: Phosphate binders, malnutrition, diarrhea, etc.
2. Transcellular shifts: Insulin, respiratory alkalosis, glucose loading, diabetic ketoacidosis, etc.
3. Renal wasting.
4. Phosphate binding agents like aluminum-containing compounds can inhibit absorption of phosphate in upper GI tract and promote phosphate depletion.
5. β-receptor agonists can shift PO_4 into cells and promote hyperphosphatemia.

Manifestations

Anorexia, myopathy, arthralgia, irritability, confusion, convulsion. Rhabdomyolysis, hemolysis in severe cases.

Hypophosphatemia can impair oxidative energy production in cells and thus adversely affect the cardiac output (reduced cardiac output) hemoglobin (hemolysis) and oxyhemoglobin dissociation (shifting of oxyhemoglobin curve to the left).

- Low phosphate levels are possible without clinical manifestations.

Treatment

1. IV phosphate replacement, if severe
2. Oral phosphate supplements
3. Correct magnesium deficit, if present
4. Treat vitamin D-deficiency, if present.

Acid-base Disturbances

The normal pH of extracellular fluid ranges from 7.36 – 7.44. Acidemia signifies a blood pH below this range and alkalemia above that range. Acidosis is a condition that leads to acidemia if there is no compensation.

Acidosis and acidemia are often regarded as same though it is not strictly true. Alkalosis and alkalemia are defined in a similar manner.

Metabolic Acidosis

It denotes a fall in blood pH and excessive acidity of body fluids secondary to an increase in acids other than carbonic acid. There may be a primary gain of acid or loss of bicarbonate from ECF. Blood pH is less than 7.35 and HCO_3^- concentration is less than 20 mEq/L.

Causes

1. Inadequate tissue oxygenation (lactic acidosis).
2. Diabetic ketoacidosis and starvation ketoacidosis.
3. Renal failure.
4. Hepatic failure.
5. Shock and cardiac arrest.
6. Increased skeletal muscle activity. Malignant hyperthermia.
7. Cyanide poisoning, carbon monoxide poisoning, and aspirin poisoning.
8. Salicylate, ethylene glycol, and methyl alcohol poisoning.
9. Diarrhea, pancreatic fistula, and renal tubular acidosis.
10. Ammonium chloride therapy.

Clinical Manifestations

1. Headache, drowsiness, confusion, and coma.
2. Decreased cardiac function and dysrhythmia.
3. Shock, tissue hypoxia, vasodilation and hypotension.
4. Dyspnea and tachypnea.
5. Nausea and vomiting.

Laboratory Investigations

1. pH less than 7.35.

2. PaCO$_2$ usually normal, may be decreased with compensation.
3. HCO$_3$ less than 20 mEq/L.
4. Anion gap may be normal or increased depending on etiology.
5. Serum potassium may be normal or little increased.

Prevention

1. Cardiac output and tissue perfusion should be maintained.
2. Urinary output should be within normal range.
3. Monitor electrolyte and acid-base status in susceptible subjects.

Treatment

1. Treat the underlying cause of metabolic acidosis. Ensure adequate cardiac output, perfusion pressure, and tissue oxygen delivery.
2. IV administration of sodium bicarbonate to raise pH to more than 7.2 and bicarbonate level to more than 15 mmol/L. Rapid correction is not recommended.
3. Cardiopulmonary status, fluid and electrolyte balance, and neurologic and neuromuscular status should be closely assessed.

Metabolic Alkalosis

It signifies a rise in pH (excessive alkalinity of body fluids) from nonrespiratory causes. There is either a gain in bicarbonate or a loss of acid from the ECF.

Causes

1. Fluid loss from upper gastrointestinal tract, persistent vomiting as in case of pyloric stenosis, nasogastric suctioning.

2. Diuretic therapy.
3. Alkali administration.
4. Hypovolemia.
5. Hyperaldosteronism.
6. Chloride-wasting diarrhea.
7. Corticosteroid therapy.
8. Metabolism of lactate in lactated Ringer's solution, citrate in stored blood or acetate in hyperalimentation solution may cause metabolic alkalosis.

Clinical Manifestations

1. History of vomiting and use of diuretics.
2. Neuromuscular irritability—Depressed respiration.
3. Muscle cramps.
4. Tetany due to direct effect of hydrogen ion concentration and low ionized plasma calcium.
5. Muscle weakness.
6. Cardiac dysrhythmias.

Laboratory Investigations

1. Blood pH more than 7.45.
2. $PaCO_2$ may be normal or decreased in compensation. Total buffer base is high, positive base excess.
3. HCO_3 more than 26–30 mEq/L.
4. Serum potassium and chloride decreased.

Management

1. Treat the underlying cause of metabolic alkalosis.
2. Correct intravascular volume depletion.
3. Replace chloride, sodium, and potassium.
4. Monitoring of fluid and electrolyte balance and acid-base status is essential.
5. Ammonium chloride may be indicated.

6. Acetazolamide IV may be helpful to increase renal excretion of bicarbonate.
7. In cases of chronic potassium depletion, potassium should be given but with extreme caution.
8. In cases with increased loss of hydrogen ions from gastric secretion, infusion of saline may be needed with supplementation of potassium.

Respiratory Acidosis

It refers a fall in pH resulting from a rise in the $PaCO_2$ from respiratory causes.

Causes

1. Drug-induced depression of alveolar ventilation—Narcotic overdose.
2. Disorders of neuromuscular function.
3. Intrinsic lung disease.
4. Increased metabolic production of carbon dioxide, hyperthermia, hyperalimentation, hypermetabolic states.

Clinical Manifestations

1. Mental impairment, unconsciousness, and coma. Cerebral blood flow and CSF pressure increased.
2. Peripheral vasodilation.
3. Myocardial depression.
4. In initial stage, sympathetic overactivity, blood pressure may rise, warm skin, dilated engorged veins, bounding pulse—Cardiac dysrhythmias.
5. At later stage, circulatory collapse.

Laboratory Investigations

1. Blood pH below 7.35.

2. Arterial PCO_2 is above 45 mmHg.
3. Plasma bicarbonate high.
4. Total buffer base, base excess, standard bicarbonate—Normal.

Management

1. Treat the underlying cause of respiratory acidosis.
2. Correct hypoventilation—Adequate oxygenation.
3. Assisted/controlled ventilation—IPPV.
4. Adequate oxygenation.
5. Rapid lowering of chronically elevated $PaCO_2$ may decrease body carbon dioxide more rapidly and may lead to metabolic alkalosis manifesting neuromuscular irritability and seizures.
6. During anesthesia, carbon dioxide absorber should be used. Misuse of muscle relaxants, central depressant drugs and narcotic analgesics should be avoided.

Respiratory Alkalosis

It signifies excessive alkalinity and a rise in pH due to a lowering of the $PaCO_2$.

Causes

1. Iatrogenic hyperventilation of lungs. Excessive artificial ventilation.
2. Decreased barometric pressure. Patients working at high temperature or at high altitude.
3. Arterial hypoxemia.
4. Hysteria.
5. Central nervous system injury, dysfunction of respiratory centers in pons and medulla.
6. Pregnancy.

7. Salicylate poisoning.
8. Cirrhosis of liver.
9. Hypothermia due to decreased metabolic production of CO_2.

Clinical Manifestations

1. Euphoria, analgesia to some extent. Paresthesia and muscle weakness.
2. Peripheral vasoconstriction may lead to pallor. Deep rapid breathing—Tachycardia.
3. Tetany—Muscle cramps.
4. Convulsion.
5. Coma.
6. Respiratory arrest.

Laboratory Investigations

1. Blood pH is high, more than 7.45.
2. Blood $PaCO_2$ less than 35 mmHg and plasma bicarbonate less than 22 mEq/L.
3. Total buffer base, base excess and standard bicarbonate—Normal.
4. Hypokalemia.
5. Hypochloremia.

Management

1. Treat the underlying cause responsible for alveolar hyperventilation.
2. Careful adequate ventilation, avoid hyperventilation.
3. Active treatment with inhalation of carbon dioxide may prove useful.
4. Treat hypokalemia and hypochloremia.

5. Monitor arterial blood gas analysis frequently.
6. In patients with ventilatory support, overventilation should be avoided. Patients should have appropriate setting of rate and volume as dictated by arterial blood gas analysis. Patients manifesting neuromuscular irritability may benefit from decreasing the minute ventilation and increasing dead space ventilation.

Chapter 11

Miscellaneous

Disseminated Intravascular Coagulation

Disseminated intravascular coagulation (DIC) is a type of acute hemostatic failure, often characterized by uncontrolled activation of the coagulation system with consumption of platelets and procoagulants causing a paradoxic coexistence of both thrombosis and hemorrhage. It is often designated as diffuse intravascular coagulation or consumption coagulopathy or defibrination syndrome.

Pathophysiology

Normally coagulation and fibrinolysis are in a state of dynamic equilibrium. In DIC trauma or triggering agents pathologically activate the normal coagulation mechanism and cause intravascular coagulation. The usual equilibrium between coagulation and fibrinolysis is disturbed and the fibrinolytic system is actuated by the strong stimulus of activator release causing secondary fibrinolysis and subsequent bleeding. Thrombin and fibrin are simultaneously active at the site of fibrin formation. Excess clotting also causes consumption of clotting factors and platelets and the blood loses its ability to clot.

As a result, bleeding occurs at multiple sites throughout the body. Thus, different organ systems particularly the kidneys, lungs, central nervous system are often affected with the risk of microemboli.

1. Triggering agents may be either direct or indirect. Direct triggers are tissue thromboplastin, proteolytic enzymes like snake venom or lysozomal enzymes. Indirect triggers are mostly endotoxin and immune complexes and they need on interaction with other mediators like white cells, platelets or endothelial cells to produce sufficient stimulus for acute hemostatic failure.
2. Intravascular coagulation may remain in compensated form but surgery or trauma may enhance or convert it to an uncompensated state with subsequent bleeding. In severe cases, the patient's blood may be completely incoagulable.

Causes of DIC

1. Tissue injury, burns, massive trauma, crush injury, and severe intracranial damage.
2. Surgical causes: Surgery of thyroid, prostate, lungs, cardiopulmonary bypass, and extensive surgery.
3. Obstetric causes: Amniotic fluid embolism, abruptio placentae, retained placentae, placental infarct, abortion, and miscarriage.
4. Malignant conditions: Leukemia, neuroblastoma, carcinomatosis, cancer of prostate, lungs, pancreas, and stomach.
5. Sepsis/infection: Gram-positive and gram-negative infections, acute viral conditions, and septicemia.
6. Acute hemolytic conditions: Mismatched blood transfusion, massive blood transfusion, snake bite, drowning, malaria, and hemolytic uremic syndrome.

7. Prolonged shock: Severe hypoxia, and lactic acidosis.
8. Liver diseases: Fulminant hepatitis, cirrhosis of liver, and trauma.
9. Possible immune diseases: Disseminated lupus erythematosus.
10. Miscellaneous conditions: Thrombocytopenic purpura, giant hemangioma, fat embolism, heat stroke, malignant hyperthermia, adult respiratory distress syndrome (ARDS), vascular malformations, and sickle cell crisis.

Clinical Features

1. Hemorrhagic manifestations:
   a. Petechial hemorrhages, purpura, and ecchymosis.
   b. Gingivial or scleral hemorrhages.
   c. Hematuria, hematemesis, hemoptysis, melena.
   d. Excessive abnormal bleeding from different sites; may be gastrointestinal, from surgical wound, from ears, nose, vagina, rectum, IV needle insertion sites, etc.
   e. Hypotension and peripheral circulatory failure.
   f. Profound acidosis, anemia, hypoxia, circulatory failure, weakness, dyspnea, etc.
   g. Respiratory failure and shock lung syndrome.
2. Thrombotic manifestations:
   a. It depends on underlying cause and degree of organ involvement. Confusion and chest pain may occur.
   b. Oliguria.
   c. Cyanosis.
   d. Circulatory failure, cool extremities, weak or absent pulses, and low blood pressure.
   e. Coma due to intravascular coagulation in brain.
   f. Thrombosis in veins or arteries may occur.

Diagnosis

There is no specific diagnostic test for DIC. Some rapid and simple tests may have a good diagnostic value. Appropriate examination of organ suspected of causing the disorder should be performed.

1. Platelet count is low.
2. Clotting factors are low.
3. Fibrinogen content is low.
4. Bleeding time is increased.
5. Prothrombin time is increased. Thrombin clotting time is increased.
6. Level of fibrin degradation products is increased.
7. Partial thromboplastin time is increased.
8. Serum creatine phosphokinase is increased.
9. Serum lactate level is increased.
10. Other sophisticated tests such as thrombin time, factor V and VIII assay, estimation of factor VIII antigen, plasminogen, etc. may also be done. But these are time-consuming investigations and may not help much in acute clinical conditions.

Management

1. Treatment of the underlying condition is most vital:
   a. Hypoxia and acidosis should be corrected in patients with shock. Adequate oxygenation and fluid replacement are essential. Tissue perfusion should be improved.
   b. Antibiotics in patients with infection and septicemia.
   c. Surgical drainage in abscesses.
   d. Resection in case of tumor or aneurysm.
   e. Bleeding may be controlled by mechanical means.
2. Specific therapy for DIC is indicated only in cases with serious hemorrhage or thrombotic complications.

Both anticoagulant and factor replacement therapy may be dangerous in the setting of DIC and should be used with great caution.
3. Replacement therapy with fresh blood, fresh frozen plasma, fibrinogen concentrate and platelet concentrate may be indicated only when the cause of DIC is reduced or removed, otherwise these will increase the degree of intravascular coagulation.
4. Anticoagulant therapy with heparin in such cases is most controversial. Heparin inhibits the formation of new clots that will slow down the consumption factors. It prevents thrombus formation and extension of existing thrombi. But it should not be used in cases with bleeding. Heparin is not helpful in sepsis.
5. Corticosteroids are also used in the management of DIC. But its exact role is not yet clear. It has α-blocking action and protects the patients against endotoxic shock.
6. Antifibrinolytic therapy: In DIC secondary hyperfibrinolysis is common. It is mostly protective as it aids to maintain microcirculation in vital organs. Many times it needs no treatment. However, it may be effectively treated with epsilon aminocaproic acid which interrupts the fibrinolytic process through inhibition of plasmin. It should be given continuously when the cause of DIC is detected and effectively controlled.

Acute Pancreatitis

Acute pancreatic inflammation is a serious clinical condition with high mortality due to multiple system failure. Management is mostly difficult and often controversial.

Causes

1. Excessive alcohol consumption.
2. Cholelithiasis, gallbladder disease. Acute pancreatitis may accompany any form of acute hepatic necrosis.
3. Idiopathic.
4. Other factors may include trauma, abdominal surgery, viral infection, hyperparathyroidism, hyperlipoproteinemias, scorpion stings, some drugs like thiazide diuretics, oral contraceptives, isoniazid, frusemide, azathioprine, sulfonamides, etc. penetrating peptic ulcer, cardiopulmonary bypass, etc.

Pathophysiology

1. In acute inflammation of pancreas initially there is conversion of trypsinogen to activated trypsin which then converts pancreatic proenzymes to active enzymes, converts kallikreinogen to kallikrein and activates thrombolytic and thrombotic factors.
2. Trypsin and chymotrypsin digest proteins and may damage blood vessels.
3. Fat necrosis may occur due to lipase and phospholipase.
4. Autodigestion of pancreas with vascular damage, edema, hemorrhage and necrosis. Inflammation may extend to other viscera and peritoneum.
5. Kallikrein is converted to bradykinin and kallidin resulting vasodilation, increased capillary permeability, etc.
6. Thrombolytic and thrombotic factors may promote the development of DIC.
7. Pancreatitis may have three stages.
    a. Acute edematous pancreatitis—Interstitial edema, dilated capillaries and lymphatics.
    b. Necrotising pancreatitis—Acinar cell death, necrosis of adjoining fatty tissue.

c. Hemorrhagic pancreatitis—Hemorrhage within the pancreas and surrounding tissues.

Clinical Features

1. Severe epigastric pain, sudden onset, may radiate to back, chest, flanks, and lower abdomen intensified in supine position.
2. Nausea, vomiting, hiccup, anxiety, and confusion.
3. Tachycardia, tachypnea, and hypotension.
4. Cool, pale, and clammy skin.
5. Abdomen usually soft. Intestinal ileus.
6. Oliguria.
7. Coma.
8. A hemorrhagic discoloration may be seen in flanks or near umbilicus in cases of retroperitoneal hemorrhage.
9. Pleural effusion.

Investigations

1. Serum amylase, lipase—Increased.
2. Serum SGOT, SGPT, LDH—Increased.
3. Serum immunoreactive trypsinogen/trypsin—Increased.
4. Serum bilirubin may be increased.
5. Serum triglycerides—Increased.
6. Blood sugar increased.
7. Blood urea and nitrogen—Increased.
8. Serum calcium and albumin—Decreased. Hypocalcemia.
9. Total blood count, Hb%, hematocrit, coagulation studies may have to be done.
10. Plain X-ray of abdomen.
11. Chest X-ray.
12. Abdomen ultrasound.
13. CT scan abdomen.

14. Urine amylase/creatinine clearance ratio. It is increased to more than 4%.

Management

1. Supportive measures:
   a. Bed rest.
   b. Adequate fluid and electrolyte balance.
   c. Monitoring of vital signs.
   d. CVP monitoring.
   e. Insertion of indwelling urinary catheter.
   f. Insertion of a nasogastric tube and suction.
   g. Care for nutrition.
2. Drug therapy:
   a. Pain relief: Opioid analgesics—Pethidine.
   b. Fluid management: Maintenance of adequate circulating blood volume is mandatory. Intake output chart monitoring is vital. Lactated Ringer's solution may be used. Human albumin expands blood volume and raises serum protein levels. Whole blood or plasma may also be indicated. Metabolic acidosis needs correction.
   c. Hypocalcemia is common and should be corrected with IV calcium gluconate.
   d. Blood glucose level should be monitored and there is tendency to develop hyperglycemia. Insulin may be needed.
   e. Hypermagnesemia, if present should be corrected.
   f. Antibiotics: Broad-spectrum antibiotics may be needed, if infection is present. Culture sensitivity test is helpful.
   g. Anticholinergics may have some benefit in such cases.
   h. Cimetidine, antacids may also help to lessen gastric acidity and to prevent gastric bleeding.

i. Surgery is indicated in selected cases as:
   i. Bile duct obstruction and gallstones.
   ii. Pancreatic abscess.
   iii. Life-threatening hemorrhagic pancreatitis.
  j. Treatable causes of acute pancreatitis should be identified and treated.
  k. Parenteral nutrition.
  l. Peritoneal lavage/dialysis may have some role.

Complications

1. Gastrointestinal complications: Pancreatic abscess, pancreatic fistula, pseudocyst, ascites, acute cholangitis, acute intra-abdominal hemorrhage, intestinal obstruction, peritonitis, necrosis of viscera, perforation or fistula formation, etc.
2. Pulmonary complications: Pneumonitis, pleural effusion, atelectasis, adult respiratory distress syndrome (ARDS).
3. Cardiovascular complications: Shock, pericardial effusion, and circulatory failure.
4. Metabolic complications: Hyperglycemia, hypocalcemia, hypomagnesemia, hypertriglyceridemia.
5. Fat necrosis in different organs: Arthritis.
6. Disseminated intravascular coagulation (DIC).
7. Gram-negative septicemia.
8. Renal failure.
9. Respiratory failure.
10. Hepatic failure.

Drowning

Drowning is a common incident in our country and many times it needs careful management in intensive care units. Immediate resuscitation should be done by the rescuer following taking out the patient from water. Immediate resuscitation should include the usual illness of the basic life support measures such as:

1. Clear the airway.
2. Start breathing by mouth-to-mouth method.
3. Commence external cardiac massage.

With all these maneuvers the patient should be brought to hospital to provide advanced cardiac life support.

Pathophysiology

1. Hypoxemia due to intrapulmonary shunting related to water-filled alveoli and alveolar collapse secondary to inactivated surfactant.
2. Acidosis: Metabolic acidosis is mostly due to tissue hypoxia. Respiratory acidosis may also occur.
3. Fresh water aspiration causes hypervolemia, hemodilution, hemolysis, hemoglobinuria, hyperkalemia. Sodium and chloride levels decrease.
4. Salt water aspiration causes hypovolemia and hemoconcentration. Electrolyte changes include increased level of sodium, chloride, and potassium.
5. Mortality and morbidity are mostly related to the degree of pulmonary injury and cerebral hypoxia.

Management

1. Advanced cardiac life support.
2. Clear the airway. Maintain the patent airway.
3. Endotracheal intubation. IPPV with 100% oxygen. Continuous positive airway pressure (CPAP) or positive end-expiratory pressure (PEEP) is helpful.
4. Isotonic saline or Ringer's lactate solution. IV infusion. Fluid requirement should be monitored by CVP and pulmonary artery pressure.
5. Sodium bicarbonate IV to treat metabolic acidosis.

6. Gastric intubation to empty the stomach.
7. Bronchodilators to treat bronchospasm.
8. Bronchoscopic suction to remove aspirated particulate matter.
9. Correction of cardiac dysrhythmias.
10. Steroids may be effective in treating pulmonary injury.
11. Antibiotics to treat pulmonary infection.
12. Cerebral edema needs vigorous treatment. Fluid restriction, hyperventilation, osmotic diuretics, frusemide, and steroids, etc.
13. Hypothermia may occur. Slow rewarming may have to be done. Body temperature should be monitored.
14. Shock: Cautious fluid and volume replacement, vasopressors, steroids.
15. Associated other injuries, if present, need careful attention.

Complications

1. Aspiration pneumonitis, bacterial pneumonia, and ARDS.
2. Anoxic encephalopathy, and cerebral edema.
3. Cardiac arrhythmias.
4. Hypotension and shock.
5. Hypothermia.
6. Hemolysis.
7. Acute renal failure.
8. DIC.

Total Spinal Anesthesia

Total spinal anesthesia is the term used to describe an undesired production of excessive cephalad spread of local anesthetics in cerebrospinal fluid.

Causes

1. Excessive doses of local anesthetics in subarachnoid space during spinal anesthesia.
2. Inadvertent dural puncture during injection of an epidural anesthetic.
3. Misplacement of an epidural catheter into subarachnoid space and subsequent subarachnoid injection of local anesthetic drug.

Clinical Manifestations

These may develop very rapidly following inadvertent injection of massive local anesthetic drug in subarachnoid space.

1. Difficulty in breathing, and apnea.
2. Nausea, vomiting, and agitation.
3. Profound hypotension, and bradycardia.
4. Unresponsiveness—Dilated pupils.
5. Respiratory arrest.
6. Cardiac arrest.

Management

1. It is a serious condition, call for help. Resuscitative equipment and medication should be available.
2. Endotracheal intubation. Adequate ventilation. IPPV with 100% oxygen. Avoid risks of aspiration.
3. Circulatory support. IV infusion of fluids. Vasopressors may be needed.
4. Atropine sulfate, if there is bradycardia.
5. If cardiac arrest occurs, commence CPR immediately.

Prevention

1. Proper dose of local anesthetic drug should be used.

2. Dural puncture must be avoided in cases of epidural anesthesia. Aspiration should be done prior to each local anesthetic injection.
3. For safety, a small test dose should be given and judged.
4. Use dilute solutions of local anesthetics.
5. Placement of epidural catheter must be judged in correct position before injecting the drug.
6. Monitor the patients carefully following spinal/epidural block.

Complications

1. Aspiration of gastric contents. Aspiration pneumonitis.
2. Severe hypoxemia and hypercarbia.
3. Circulatory collapse.
4. Cerebral ischemia and cerebral edema.
5. Myocardial ischemia and myocardial infarction.

Transfusion Reactions

Blood and blood products are being widely used in medical practice. These are mostly lifesaving but can cause adverse reactions and even endanger life. Every attempt should be made to reduce such reactions to the minimum.

Indications for Blood Transfusion

1. **Volume replacement**: Blood loss should be replaced by blood, but losses of 800 ml – 1000 ml in healthy individual may be safely and effectively treated with intravenous colloid solutions or dextran.
2. **Correction of anemia**: Anemia is best treated with iron, folate, vitamin B_{12} and others. But it takes much time for correction of anemia. Blood transfusion and particularly packed red blood cell may be needed for early correction as in semiurgent surgical procedures.

3. Correction of hemostatic abnormalities. For such cases fresh whole blood transfusion is needed.
4. To supply immune bodies—Blood transfusion may be beneficial in chronically ill patients.

Storage of Whole Blood can Cause Following Changes

1. Red blood corpuscles: Intracellular ATP, potassium and 2, 3 DPG reduced; gas transport function decreased; membrane lipid reduced, turns to more spherical shape with decreased deformability.
2. Plasma, potassium, ammonia, citrate, and lactic acid increased; free hemoglobin increased; vasoactive substances increased; factor V and factor VIII reduced.
3. Platelets and white blood cells: Quantity reduced, functional defects are common, reduction of labile clotting factors.
4. Formation of microaggregates.

Whole blood is usually preserved in acid citrate-dextrose (ACD) solution. The storage period is 21–28 days. Newer preservatives, citrate-phosphate-dextrose (CPD) or citrate-phosphate-double dextrose-adenine (CP2D-adenine) can prolong more efficient storage. It results in a longer shelf life upto 35 days, improves oxygen transport, decreased microaggregates formation and reduced potassium leakage.

Note

1. Increase in plasma ammonia is relatively contraindicated in patients with liver dysfunction.
2. Too microaggregates may make transfusion difficult.
3. Storage period for platelets is short about 48 hours and for white cell is only few hours.
4. No problem with long-term storage of stable plasma protein solution, concentrated human serum albumin,

fresh frozen plasma, prothrombin complex factors II, VI, IX, and X and fibrinogen.

Adverse Effects of Blood Transfusion

It may be divided into reactions that can occur immediately following transfusion and those occur in later time ranging from few days to several years.

These reactions can also be further divided into antibody-mediated and nonantibody-mediated effects.

A. Immediate transfusion reactions

a. Antibody-mediated reactions:
 1. Acute hemolytic transfusion reaction.
 2. *Simple febrile reactions*: These are manifested by rigor, fever, nausea and vomiting. This is mostly due to the presence of white cell antigens, gram-negative endotoxin and faulty aseptic measures.
    Management: Stop transfusion and antipyretics.
 3. *Allergic manifestations*: These are mostly due to response to transfused antigens and manifested with skin rashes, rigor, hypotension and even bronchospasm. Antihistamics may be helpful for prevention and treatment.
 4. *Anaphylactic reaction*: It is due to antigen-antibody reaction releasing vasoactive and smooth muscle reactive mediators manifested by flushing, hypotension, shock laryngeal/ pulmonary edema, bronchospasm, etc.
    Management: Stop transfusion. 100% oxygenation and ventilation. IV fluids, adrenaline, broncho dilators, and cardiopulmonary resuscitation.
 5. Transfusion-related acute lung injury. Donor WBC antibodies reacts with recipient WBC and

produce white cell aggregates which are trapped in lung vasculature causing increased vascular permeability. Clinical features include respiratory distress, dyspnea, fever, cyanosis, hypotension, low pulmonary wedge pressure, and pulmonary infiltrates on chest X-ray.

Management: Stop transfusion, steroids, and IPPV with 100% oxygen.

b. Nonantibody-mediated reactions:
   1. *Overloading of circulation*: It is due to excessive or too rapid transfusion. Congestive cardiac failure and pulmonary edema can occur.

      Clinical manifestations: Tachycardia, dyspnea, cough, cyanosis, engorged neck veins, hypertension/hypotension, and elevated CVP.

      Management: Stop transfusion. IPPV, frusemide, dopamine to improve cardiac contractility.

   2. *Infection*: Gram-negative endotoxemia, septicemia. It is due to contaminated stored blood, poor sterility measures, pre-existing infection of donor, etc. Often manifested with rigor, fever, shock, disseminated intravascular coagulation, and renal failure.

      Management: Stop transfusion, IV antibiotics, IV fluids, dopamine, and phenylephrine.

   3. *Citrate intoxication*: It is due to recduced ionized plasma calcium concentration, if large volumes of stored blood is transfused rapidly. Clinical features include tingling, muscle cramps, cardiac arrhythmia, prolonged QT interval on ECG, increased pulmonary capillary wedge persure, and cardiac arrest.

      Management: Stop blood transfusion, calcium administration, and supportive care.

   4. Hypothermia can occur due to rapid transfusion of cold blood. Adequate preventive measures should be taken.

5. Generalized bleeding can occur due to low content of platelets and clotting factors in stored blood.
6. Metabolic acidosis can occur due to transfusion of large volume of stored blood.
7. Ammonia content of stored blood is high so it may adversely affect the patients with liver disease.
8. Hyperkalemia can occur as red cell potassium leaks extracellularly in stored blood. Manifestations include muscle weakness, bradycardia, prolonged PR interval QRS and QT interval, Peaked T-waves, and ventricular fibrillation.

   Management: Stop transfusion, IV calcium chloride, glucose with regular insulin, and dialysis in extreme cases.
9. Air embolism can occur due to faulty apparatus or transfusion under pressure.
10. *Massive blood transfusion*: It implies transfusion of half of the calculated blood volume or more in less than 1 hour or the whole blood volume during 24 hours or less. It also implies if the 10% of blood volume is replaced in 10 minutes or less.

    This can cause certain biochemical and coagulation abnormalities in addition to large volume replacement. Moreover pre-existing shock and underlying disease and storage lesion of transfusing blood deteriorates the condition. On the whole, there are defective gas transport system of cells and high content of citrate potassium, lactic acid, and ammonia. Coagulation disorders, pulmonary microemboli, hypothermia, and adult respiratory distress syndrome can also result.

Preventive and therapeutic measures:

1. Adequate oxygenation and ventilation.
2. Blood should be as fresh as possible.

3. Blood warming device should be used.
4. Blood filler is helpful.
5. Monitor arterial blood gas analysis and serum.
6. Acidosis should be corrected.
7. For every 2 liters of blood transfuse, two units of fresh frozen plasma is advised.
8. Screening of blood coagulation studies is essential. Treat the abnormalities accordingly.
9. If DIC is present and heparin is indicated.
10. General supportive care.

Acute hemolytic transfusion reactions—

It occurs when donor RBC's antigen and recepient's plasma antibodies are incompatible. ABO mismatch occurs when the recipient receives wrong blood. It can occur due to faulty identification of patients, samples labels, and donor units.

Hemolytic transfusion reaction may be of two types:

 i. Intravascular hemolysis due to specific incompatible blood transfusion.
 ii. Extravascular nonspecific type due to transfusion of lysed blood; old, outdated overheated or frozen blood.

Manifestations include pain along the transfusion line, shaking, chills, fever, nausea, abdominal cramps, loin pain, chest pain, sweating, vasodilation and hypotension. Oliguria and renal failure can occur. Pink-red serum, hemoglobinuria, bleeding diathesis, and cardiovascular collapse may follow. Some patients can develop DIC and ARDS.

Management

1. Stop blood transfusion.
2. IV fluid infusion to maintain circulatory blood volume and urine output.

3. Remains of blood in the bottle and the fresh blood are to be sent for further investigation
4. Urine examination and blood examination.
5. Treat hypotension: IV fluids and vasopressors.
6. Frusemide and mannitol.
7. Sodium bicarbonate.
8. Maintain urine output at least 100 ml/hour.
9. Treat DIC—Platelets, fresh frozen plasma, and cryoprecipitate may be helpful. Heparin can minimize intravascular coagulation.
10. Hemodialysis in selected cases of renal failure.
11. Oxygen therapy and ventilation in cases of hypoxia.
12. General supportive care. Cooling and antipyretics in cases of pyrexia.
13. Prevention should always be tried—
    i. Identification of patients at risk.
    ii. Autotransfusion should be encouraged.
    iii. Transfusion should be given only when it is absolutely indicated.
    iv. Adequate checking of documents before transfusion is essential.
    v. Strict monitoring is essential during transfusion for early diagnosis and treatment.

B. Delayed reactions

a. Antibody-mediated delayed reactions:
   1. Delayed sensitization usually complicates future transfusion or pregnancy due to Rh factor.
   2. Delayed hemolytic transfusion reaction. Fever and anemia may appear a few days after transfusion. Jaundice and renal failure can occur.
   3. Alloimmunization to RBC, platelet, or WBC antigens.
   4. Graft vs host disease.
   5. Post-transfusion purpura.

b. Nonantibody-mediated delayed reactions:
   1. Hemosiderosis, deposition of iron in tissue is due to repeated transfusions given over many years as in cases of aplastic anemia.
   2. Some diseases may be transmitted from the donor—
      i. Malaria
      ii. Kala-azar
      iii. Syphilis.
   3. Viral hepatitis.
   4. Trypanosomiasis.
   5. Bacteremia and septicemia.
   6. AIDS.
   7. Human T lymphocites virus—Type I.

Dengue

Dengue is a viral acute febrile illness, caused by one of four serotypes of flavivirus. It is transmitted by the bite of *Aedes* mosquito infected with dengue virus. The incubation period ranges from 7–10 days. It may be in epidemic form in many parts of developing countries. Children are more susceptible. The disease is not predictable in its course and presentation. Majority patients develop mild symptoms and only few cases suffer severe dengue, often with life-threatening complications. Complications usually occur during defervescence 5th day of illness in the form of shock, bleeding, respiratory distress and encephalopathy, etc.

Manifestations

1. Sudden onset of fever, chills, severe muscle pain, joint pain, sore throat, nausea/vomiting, abdominal pain, headache, lethargy, etc.
2. Fever is usually biphasic, initial phase of 3–4 days, short remission followed by second phase of 1–2 days.

3. Neutropenia and thrombocytopenia.
4. *Rash*: It is initially evanescent followed by maculopapular, scarlatiniform, morbilliform or petechial changes during remission or second phase of fever. It first appears in extremities and then to the body.
5. *Severe dengue*: Here the disease is complicated with severe plasma leakage leading to shock, fluid accumulation in abdomen and/ or thorax, respiratory distress gastrointestinal hemorrhage, liver dysfunction, central nervous system involvement, impaired consciousness, and coma.

Investigations

A. Hematocrit is most important in identifying the degree of capillary leakage, if any, and in guiding therapy.
B. *Liver function tests*: Raised hepatic enzymes may indicate hepatic involvement.
C. X-ray of chest and abdomen may show pleural fluid or ascitic fluid.
D. Serological and antigen detection can confirm the diagnosis.

Management

1. Early detection and early management of severe dengue are most important to reduce the incidences of mortality and morbidity.
2. Strict clinical and laboratory monitoring.
3. No drug is effective against the virus. General supportive care. Antipyretics and analgesics.
4. Public health measures and community involvement are mandatory to control the epidemic.
5. Treatment of severe dengue—
    A. *Shock*: IV fluid, O_2 administration, vasopressors, Inotropes and dopamine.

B. *Bleeding*: Fresh blood transfusion, fresh frozen plasma, and cryoprecipitate transfusion.
C. Treat hypoxia and acidosis. 100% oxygenation. IPPV.
D. Fluid overload must be prevented.

   Administration of fluids, blood, etc. should be judicious. Careful monitoring of blood pressure, pulse, urine output and perfusion is helpful. Ventilator support with PEEP may be needed.
E. Treat the cardiogenic shock, arrhythmias and conduction block, if any.
F. *Encephalopathy*: Airway protection, IPPV, minimum sedation, osmotic diuretics, and anticonvulsant in cases with seizures.

Bibliography

1. Adams AP, Cashman JN. Anaesthesia. Analgesia and Intensive Care. London: Edward Arnold. 1994.
2. Baldwin KM, Garza CS, Martin RN, Sheritt S, Hanssen GA. Davis's Manual of Critical Care Therapeutics. New Delhi: Jaypee Brothers Medical Publishers (P) Ltd. 1996.
3. Campbell D, Spence AA. Anaesthetics, Resuscitation and Intensive Care. Edinburgh: Churchill Livingstone. 1978.
4. Condon RE, Decosse JJ. Surgical Care. Philadelphia: Lea and Febiger. 1980.
5. Dripps, Eckenholf, Vandam. Introduction to Anaesthesia. Philadelphia: WB Saunders Co. 1997.
6. Goba DM, Fish KJ, Howard SK. Crisis Management in Anaesthesiology. New York: Churchill Livingstone. 1994.
7. Hopkn DAB. Anaesthesia, Recovery and Intensive Care. London: English University Press 1970.
8. Kaufman L, Ginsberg R. Anaesthesia Review. New York: Churchill Livingstone. 1987; Vol. 13
9. Kirby RK, Grdvenstein N, Lobato EB, Gravein Stein JS. Clinical Anaesthesia Practice. Philadelphia: WB Saunders Company. 2002.

10. Orland MJ, Saltman RJ. Manual of Medical Therapeutics. Boston: Little Brown and Company. 1986.
11. Paul AK. Clinical Anaesthesia. Kolkata: Academic Publishers. 2002.
12. Ravin MB. Problems in Anaesthesia. Boston: Little Brown. 1981.
13. Reed AP. Clinical Cases of Anaesthesia. New York: Churchill Livingstone. 1995.
14. Stoelting RK, Diedorf SF. Handbook of Anaesthesia and Coexisting Disease. New York: Churchill Livingstone. 1995.
15. Stoelting RK, Miller RD. Basics of Anaesthesia. New York: Churchill Livingstone. 1995.

Index

A

Acid-base disturbances 186
Acidosis
    metabolic 187
    respiratory 190
Acute
    hemolytic transfusion reaction 211
    pancreatitis 198
Adrenocortical insufficiency 132
Airway burn 26
Alkalosis
    metabolic 188
    respiratory 191
Aspiration pneumonitis 20
Asthma 5

B

Bicarbonate 167
Brain death 82
Bronchitis 8

C

Cardiac
    arrest 160
    asystole 166
    tamponade 53
Cardiopulmonary resuscitation 160
Cerebrovascular accident 65
Chlordiazepoxide 151
Chlorpromazine 151
Cholinergic crisis 95
Coagulation
    diffuse intravascular 194
    disseminated intravascular 194
Coma 86
    diabetic 139
    hyperglycemic hyperosmolar nonketotic 127
    myxedemic 122
Consumption coagulopathy 194

D

Defibrillation 165
Dehydration 169
Diabetes 125
Diabetic
    ketoacidosis 125
    neuropathy 108
Dialysis 116
Diazepam 151
Disease
    chronic obstructive pulmonary 8
    liver 97
    lung 1
    renal 107
    thyroid 120

Drowning 202
Drug overdose 144

E

Edema
  acute pulmonary 39
  cerebral 66
  noncardiogenic pulmonary 1
  pulmonary 39
Electromechanical dissociation 166
Emphysema 8
Encephalopathy 103
Endocrine dysfunctions 120

F

Failure
  chronic respiratory 10
  congestive cardiac 34
  heart 35
  liver
    acute 97
    chronic 102
  renal 107
  respiratory 8
Fat embolism 11
Flail chest 27
Fluid and electrolyte balance 144
Fluid, electrolyte, and acid-base disorders 169

G

Glasgow coma scale 62
Glomerulonephritis 112

H

Heat stroke 134
Hemodialysis 116
Hemorrhage 46
Hepatic encephalopathy 103
Hepatitis 97
Hypercalcemia 172
Hyperkalemia 175
Hypernatremia 179
Hyperphosphatemia 184
Hypertensive crisis 44
Hypoadrenalism 139
Hypocalcemia 174
Hypoglycemia 130
Hypokalemia 177
Hyponatremia 181
Hypophosphatemia 185

I

Injury
  brain 61
  chest 16
  head 59
Intracranial pressure 77

J

Jaundice 98

L

Lorazepam 151

M

Malignant hyperthermia 135

Massive blood transfusion 210
Meningitis 86
Myasthenia gravis 94
Myocardial infarction 29

N

Nephritis 112
Nervous system disorders 59
Nontraumatic spinal cord disorder 94

P

Peritoneal dialysis 117
Pneumothorax 15
Poisoning
   alcohol 152
   aspirin 146
   barbiturate 145
   cocaine 156
   cyanide 155
   depletion 190
   dextropropoxyphene 150
   ethanol 152
   imipramine 148
   insecticides 151
   irritant gases 157
   lithium 149
   malathion 149
   methyl alcohol 153
   morphine 150
   narcotic 150
   organophosphorus 151
   paracetamol 147
   parathion 151
   pethidine 150
   phenobarbitone 145
   salicylate 146
   tranquilizers 151
   tricyclic antidepressants drugs 148
   with amphetamines 155
   with caustics 158
Poliomyelitis 72
Potassium
   depletion 190
   excess 179
Pulmonary embolism 10
Pure water deficiency 170

R

Renal transplantation 118
Respiratory disorders 1

S

Self-poisoning 142
Shock
   anaphylactic 46
   bacteremic 52
   cardiogenic 46
   hypovolemic 46
   neurogenic 46
Skull fractures 60
Sodium
   depletion 181
   excess 179
Spinal column injuries 91
Status
   asthmaticus 5
   epilepticus 69
Syndrome
   adult respiratory distress 1
   Guillain-Barré 84
   hepatorenal 104
   respiratory distress 1
   shock lung 1

T

Temperature illness 134
Tetanus 74
Thyroid storm 120
Thyrotoxic crisis 120
Total spinal anesthesia 204
Transfusion reactions 206
Traumatic spinal cord injury 90

U

Upper airway obstruction 24

V

Ventricular fibrillation 165

W

Water intoxication (excess) 171